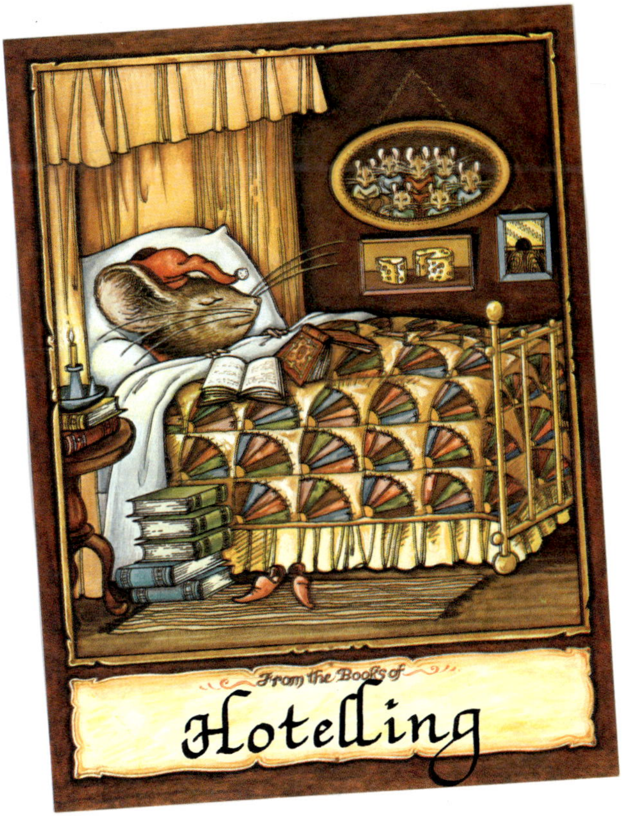
From the Books of
Hotelling

INGE J. BLEIER, R.N., B.S., M.S.
Maternity Nursing Instructor, DePaul University, Chicago.
Formerly Instructor, Maternal and Child Health Nursing,
University of Illinois; Maternity Nursing Instructor,
Michael Reese Hospital and Medical Center;
Maternity Supervisor and Instructor,
Louis A. Weiss Memorial Hospital, Chicago

workbook in

BEDSIDE MATERNITY NURSING

second edition

1974
W. B. SAUNDERS COMPANY
Philadelphia, London, Toronto

W. B. Saunders Company: West Washington Square
Philadelphia, PA 19105

12 Dyott Street
London, WC1A 1DB

833 Oxford Street
Toronto 18, Ontario

Workbook in Bedside Maternity Nursing ISBN 0-7216-1746-8

Last digit is the print number: 9 8 7 6 5 4 3 2 1

TO THE INSTRUCTOR

The new edition of this workbook was prepared to include the contemporary issues, developments, and innovations in the field of maternity nursing. Among the added topics you will find sex and the young adult; an extensive presentation of the four basic food groups, including the calories of each item listed, in order to guide the student in menu planning and teaching of nutrition; inclusion of problems facing black and adolescent couples; discussion of venereal disease; phototherapy in hyperbilirubinemia; sickle cell disease; and the updating of the abortion laws. New questions and problems relevant to our times are posed. Diagrams pertinent to regional anesthesia and other medical procedures have been included in order to clarify these procedures for the student. Responding to the numerous requests of instructors, the workbook now presents 170 multiple choice questions, which appear following the last chapter. This comprehensive examination will reveal whether the student has mastered the issues of maternity nursing and at the same time will prepare her for taking the State Board Examinations. (None of these questions are duplicates of the ones published in my book *Maternity Nursing* and its accompanying Instructor's Guide.)

As in the former edition the workbook tests medical knowledge and nursing skills, and requires the use of the behavioral sciences and interpersonal relations.

The workbook is not based on a specific textbook or definite nursing articles. For this reason applicable references include any of the contemporary maternity texts and the obstetric articles listed in the Index of Nursing Periodicals, and Briefs, published by the New York Maternity Center. I strongly advise the use of new articles and texts as they appear; these will either support the answers given in the Answer Key or update them.

Lastly, I wish to thank each instructor who offered constructive advice, for this helped immensely in the preparation of the revision of the workbook.

TO THE STUDENT

Every practitioner of maternity nursing must have at her fingertips basic knowledge that contributes toward optimum care of the new family. In the following chapters you will apply your knowledge in the various fields which constitute maternity nursing.

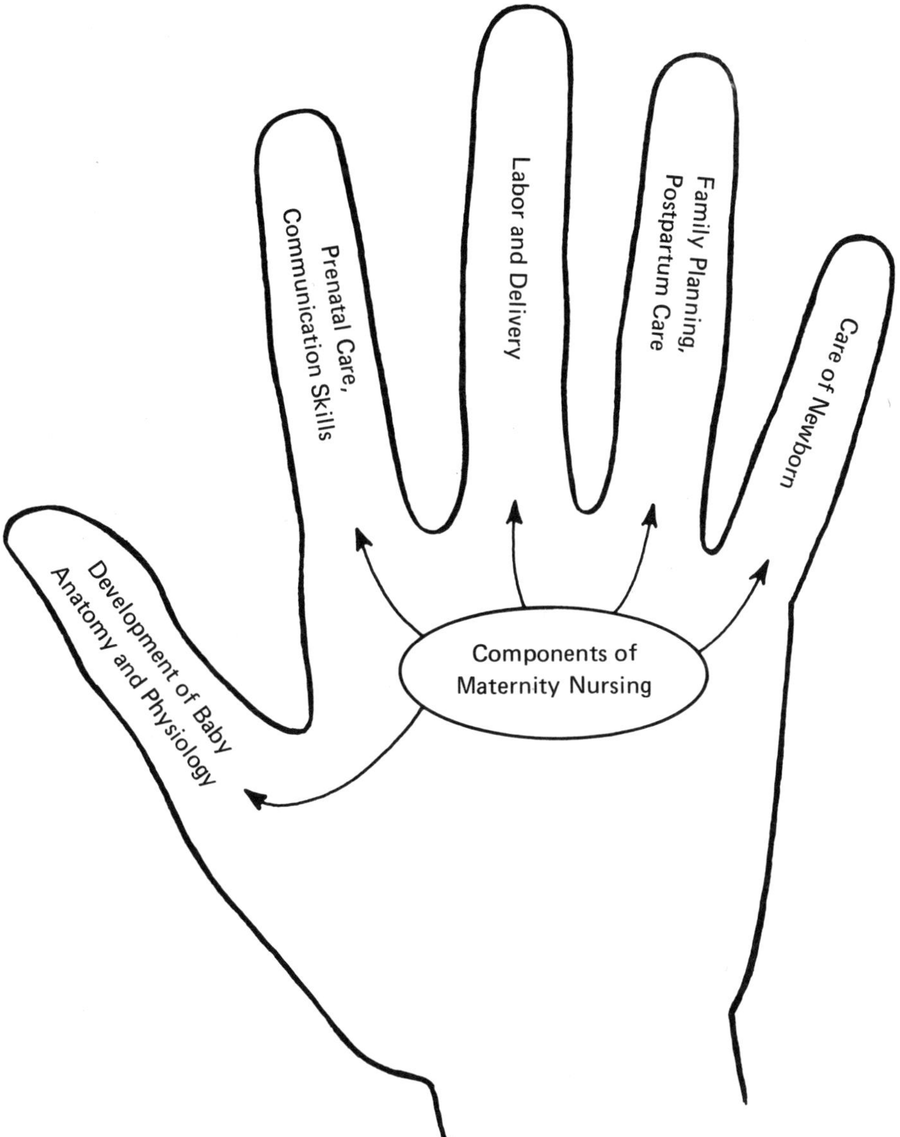

Contents

Anatomy of the Reproductive Organs and Pelvis

EXTERNAL GENITALIA

Mrs. Mary Gross, 38 years old, is expecting her first baby. She has been in labor for 18 hours and her physician expects her to deliver within four hours. Her abdominal contour reveals a full bladder. She is unable to void spontaneously. A catheterization is ordered.

You bring to her bedside a catheterization tray.

1. Now you are going to explain the procedure to Mrs. Gross. What are you actually telling her?

2. You are right-handed. In carrying out the catheterization procedure, which structures are you separating and slightly pulling up with your left hand?

(a) ________________________________

(b) ________________________________

3. The external genitalia are now exposed to you. Label them on the diagram (Figure 1).

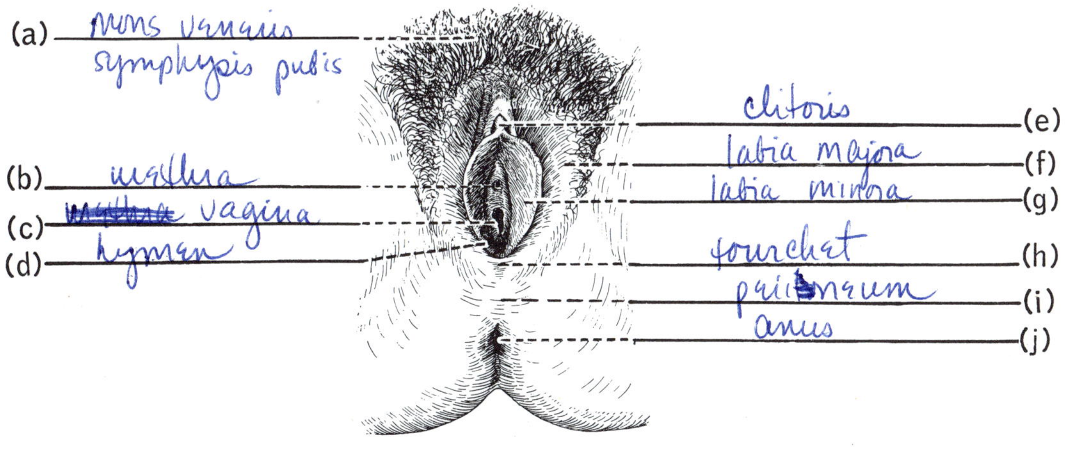

Figure 1.

4. The urinary meatus is located between the vagina

and clitoris.

5. The female urethra is approximately ________ long. How far are you going to insert the catheter?

6. What important precaution must you observe when handling and inserting the catheter?

7. If this precaution is ignored what could be the consequence for Mrs. Gross?

8. How much urine is it safe to remove from the bladder in one catheterization?

9. State the reason for not exceeding this amount.

10. The external genitalia extending from the lower vaginal orifice to

the rectum are called perineum.

It is made up of muscles into which an incision, called an episiotomy, is sometimes made at the time of delivery. The purpose for an episiotomy is to enlarge the vaginal outlet.

11. The largest vulvovaginal glands are located at the lateral margins of

the vaginal orifice. Their name is Bartholin's glands.

12. What is their function?

secrete mucoid material during sexual excitement

INTERNAL REPRODUCTIVE ORGANS

Betty Bell is a high school senior who is planning marriage two weeks following graduation. Today she is seeing the obstetrician for a premarital examination. After you finish taking Betty's history she suddenly says: "Why does the doctor need to examine me internally?"

13. How do you phrase your answer?

14. Betty says that she would like to know more about the female reproductive organs. To help you with your explanation you show her a diagram of the internal reproductive structures and identify them for her. Indicate your identification below (Figure 2).

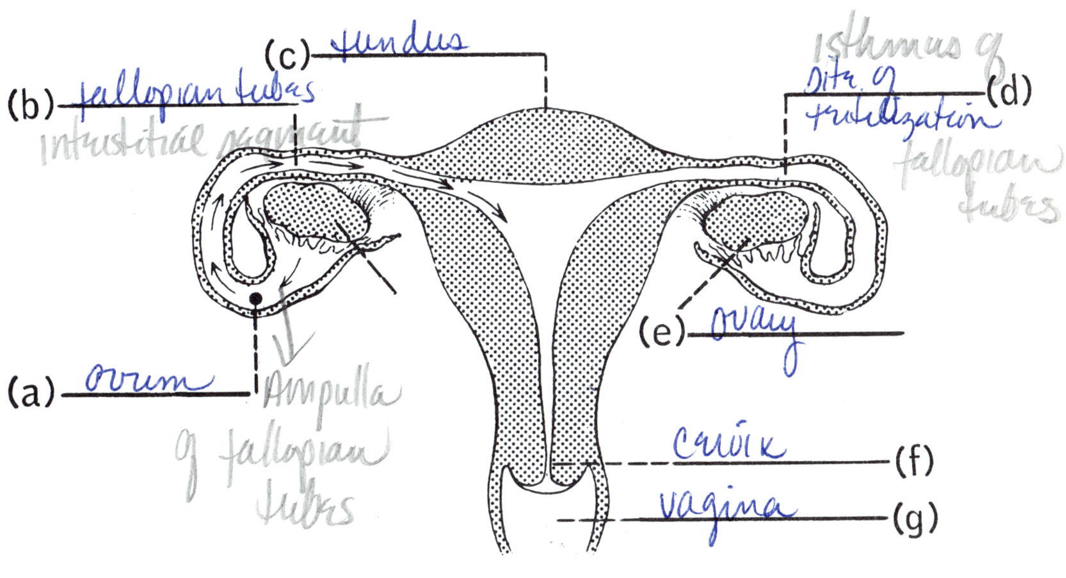

Figure 2.

To function in maternity nursing, you yourself must have more detailed knowledge of the uterus. Therefore:

15. Name the two parts of the uterus.

(a) ____

(b) ____

16. The upper section of the uterus above the entrance of the fallopian tubes is called ___fundus___________________ .

17. Label the layers of the uterine wall and the parts of the cervix on the diagram (Figure 3).

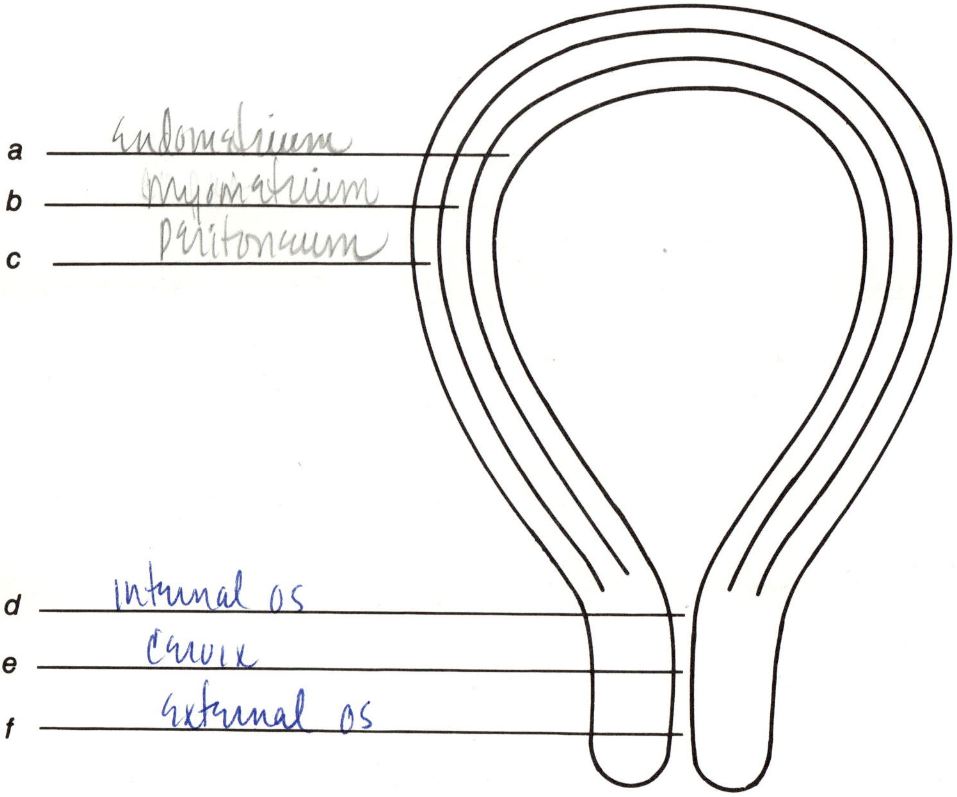

Figure 3.

THE PELVIS

18. Define the role of the pelvis in obstetrics.

19. Label the following structures on the diagram (Figure 4).

Sacrum	Pubis
Coccyx	Ischial spine
Ilium	Ischial tuberosity
Ischium	Symphysis pubis

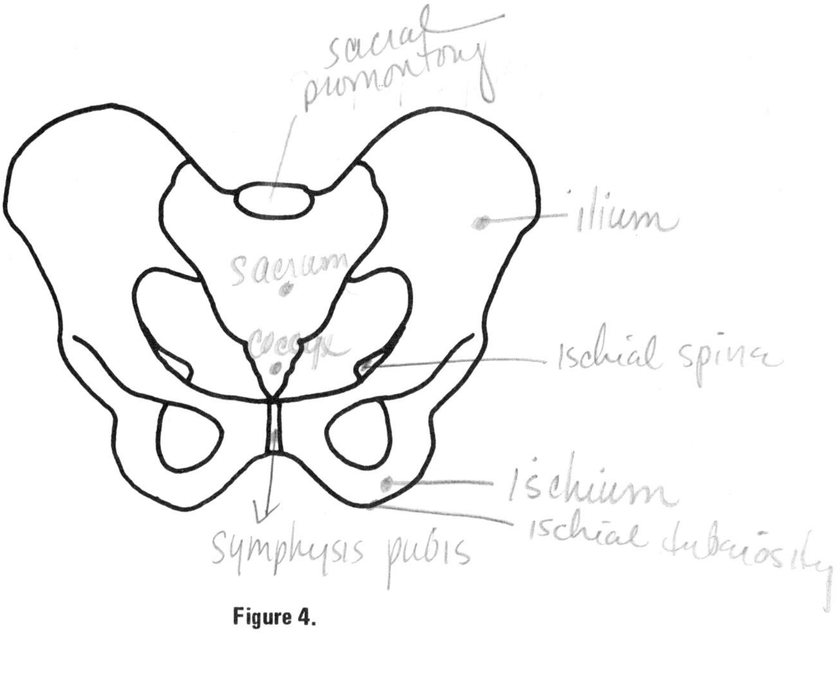

Figure 4.

20. The shortest diameter of the pelvic cavity is the distance between the posterior aspect of symphysis pubis + sacral promontory.

21. Name the three parts that make up the true pelvis.

(a) ______

(b) ______

(c) ______

22. What information can be gained from x-ray pelvimetry?

23. If x-ray pelvimetry is indicated, it is most advisable to take it during which period of pregnancy? Why?

Physiology of the Reproductive Organs

Research studies indicate that ovulation takes place about 14 days before menstruation. Therefore, the fertile time for women who flow every 28 days is halfway between menses, or about the fourteenth day. But for women who menstruate every 21 to 35 days, the ovulation time, or fertile period, will occur between the seventh and twenty-first days following the last menstruation.

1. While you talk with Betty Bell you learn that her menstruations occur regularly every 30 days. Her last menstrual period started on Tuesday, October 1, and lasted till Saturday, the fifth. (Today is Wednesday, the ninth.) On the calendar show Betty when she will probably ovulate this month. Color the day (or days) in red. With a blue pencil mark the day on which she can expect her next menstrual period (Figure 5).

2. For your own exercise encircle with a green pencil the days on which fertilization could occur.

3. Number the following stages of ovarian activity in the order of their occurrence during the menstrual cycle.

______ Degeneration of corpus luteum

______ Ovulation

______ Period during which corpus luteum is present and functioning

______ Period of follicle growth and function

4. What structure is present in the ovary:

(a) Prior to ovulation______________________________

(b) Following ovulation______________________________

OCTOBER

S	M	T	W	T	F	S
		1	2	3	4	5
6	7	8	9	10	11	12
13	14	15	16	17	18	19
20	21	22	23	24	25	26
27	28	29	30	31		

Figure 5.

5. What is the stage of endometrial development:

(a) Immediately before ovulation proliferative

(b) Following ovulation secretory

6. In what phase are the cells of the endometrium when a fertilized ovum arrives for implantation?

7. Name the two hormones secreted by the ovary.

(a) estrogen

(b) progesterone

8. Normal ovarian function requires the influence of two anterior pituitary hormones. They are the follicle-stimulating and the luteinizing hormone.

The above two hormones are referred to collectively as the pituitary gonadotropins.

9. Label the pituitary and ovarian hormones in the diagram (Figure 6).

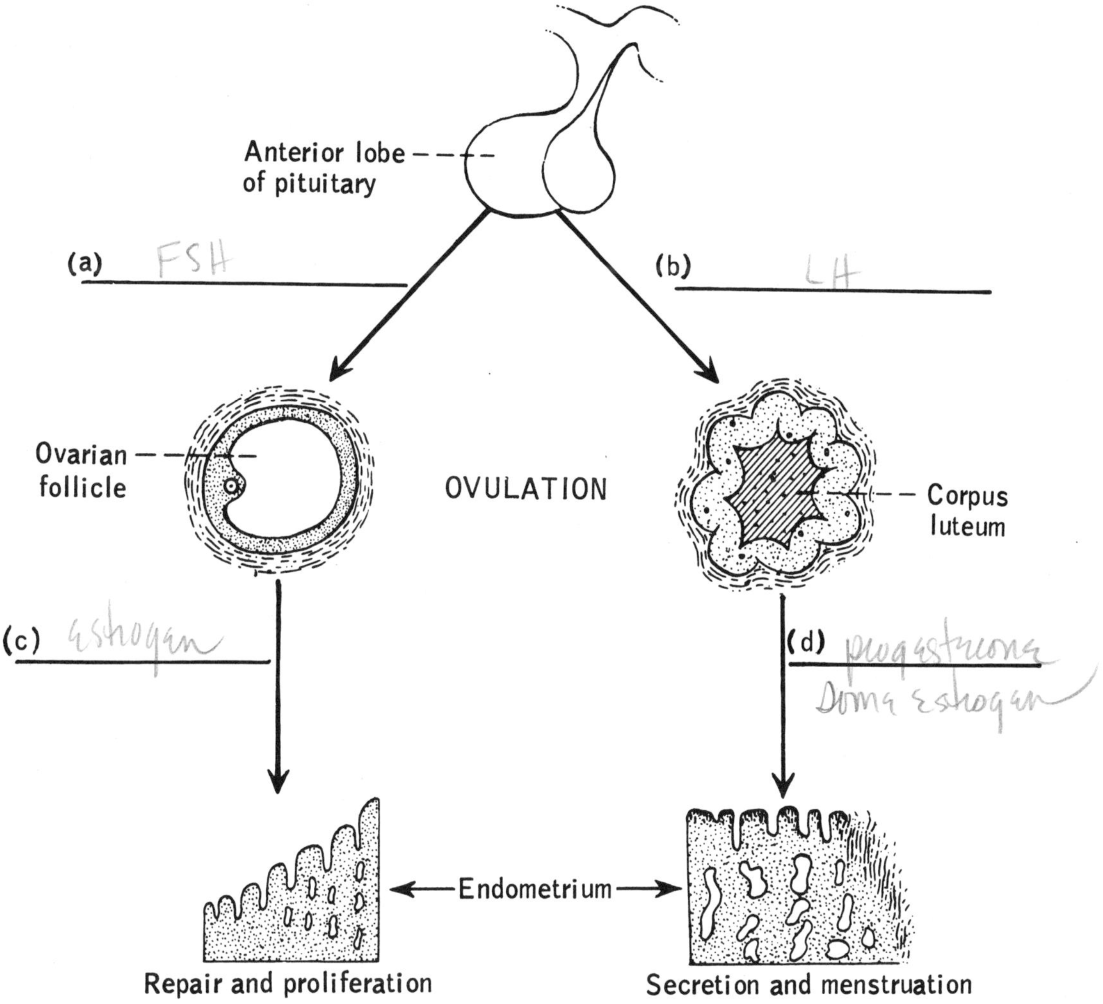
Anterior lobe of pituitary
(a) FSH
(b) LH
Ovarian follicle
OVULATION
Corpus luteum
(c)
(d)
Endometrium
Repair and proliferation
Secretion and menstruation

Figure 6.

Sex and the Young Adult

Inasmuch as we are counseling younger people than a decade ago, and because their attitudes are different from those of past generations, this description of the current approaches in sexual counseling is presented.

It is generally acknowledged that many American college students are entering into sexual relationships today more readily than did their counterparts in earlier generations. This change in sexual behavior has been coming on for a long time; liberalization has been more or less continuous since the Victorian era. But a development that has come only recently, particularly since the mid '60s, is the great increase in the openness with which young people pursue their sexual lives and talk about them.

Because of this new openness, adults involved with people of college age—parents, educators, and others—are much more aware of the prevailing patterns of sexual behavior than was true formerly. As a consequence, many are more concerned about sex-related problems than was the case in those eras when overt sexual activity was less evident, even if not less prevalent.

One thing to be said for the new openness is that it makes possible the freer discussion of sex-related problems. And this is all to the good, because, as anyone who lives and works with college students today is aware, they may have overcome many of their own inhibitions and have won liberal concessions from society, but, like other human beings, they have not discovered a foolproof way to enter into sexual relationships without involving themselves in serious and complex emotional situations.

No one—including the college physician or psychologist—can claim to be an expert in the whole broad area of youth and sex, but those of us who spend our time talking and working with college students do have firsthand access to information not generally available.

Even to approach an understanding of young people's current sexual attitudes, it is necessary to recognize that their prevalent belief—and one which has gained ascendancy rather recently—is that feeling is at least as sound a basis for behavior as is logical thinking. To many, actions stemming from feelings need no apology. Since sex is always based on feeling or is the expression of feeling (sometimes of several different feelings), it must in itself be good. This attitude, crystallized during the so-called "youth revolution" of recent years, is in sharp contrast to the older conviction that feelings were not to be trusted as much as reason in the formulation of bases for behavior and standards of values. Though I have stated the position in its extreme form, the general attitude of "belief in feeling" has markedly diminished young people's adherence to older codes of behavior based purely on reason or tradition.

Equally strong among young people today is the emphasis on absolute honesty (meaning frankness and openness as well as truthfulness) in relationships, including sexual ones. A relationship which is honest, loving and caring, both emotionally and physically, is considered desirable, something one wants for oneself and for those one cares about. And just as it is essential to be honest with one's partner, so it is important to be honest (and open) with the rest of the world about one's actions and about the fact that those actions are based on genuine feelings and not on respect for appearances. Behaving one way for the sake of appearances or because of the reaction of one's elders, when you actually feel like (and therefore believe in) doing something else, is widely regarded as hypocritical; and hypocrisy, rather than, say, premarital sex, has become the real sin in the eyes of many young people.

This concern for honesty in human relations is at least partly a reflection of young people's disillusionment with the increasingly impersonal nature of our society and its tendency to rely on appearances rather than fundamental values. They resent and consider hypocritical those huge corporations preoccupied with their own sheer size and growth, the bureaucratic organizations strangling themselves and their clients in red tape, and the consequent reduction of individuals from names to numbers. According to their view, society needs to be more open and sincere, while individuals must retain and protect their humanness by being more natural in their behavior.

In terms of sex, young people are aware that premarital intercourse, marital infidelity, and sexual deviation have long been widespread in our society, but not honestly acknowledged. Often they regard such a denial of reality as hypocrisy and refuse to give lip service to codes of behavior which clearly, and in their view inevitably, are being widely flouted. They believe that rules should respect reality, should take into account what real people are really doing, should regulate the game that is actually being played and not some game that someone wishes were being played.

This is, of course, in direct opposition to the view of earlier generations that rules encouraged high standards of behavior by challenging people to attempt to live up to them. Thus, traditionalists often argue that although premarital sex and extramarital sex are going on, it would be better if they were not, and that they may be encouraged by the relaxation of rules against them, even though many persons pay only lip service to those rules.

Even if young people today accepted the traditional moral evaluations of sexual practices, they would still oppose attempts to upgrade behavior by pretending, through idealized standards, that human behavior is better than it is. And, of course, many young people do not accept the old moral evaluations. Many of them today—probably a majority—feel that premarital sex is not only acceptable but also desirable under some circumstances, notably when two people love each other. Laws or rules established by a college or any other institution in an effort to eliminate premarital sex will not change that attitude, and can influence actual behavior only to the minimal extent that such laws or rules are enforceable. Indeed, they will be counterproductive insofar as they will be regarded as encouraging dishonesty rather than reinforcing honesty, and thus will lessen respect for the institution promulgating them.

Another factor contributing to the new openness about sexual conduct is the notable increase in informality, spontaneity, and directness of approach in all areas of young people's behavior. Combined with the increased respect for feeling, this new life style results in a much freer, more casual attitude toward sex. Relationships are established much more easily and readily, including sexual relationships. Spontaneous activities among young people who simply enjoy each other's company have largely replaced the formal dating of yesterday. Invitations are extended casually and plans made mutually instead of on a rigid man-invites-woman basis, and easy friendship and companionship, which in an earlier day sometimes were lost in formalities, have come into their own.

It is probably not surprising, then, that many (but not all) young people of college age feel that a relationship will, indeed probably should, include sexual intercourse if the two people involved are genuinely fond of each other. Some go even further and say that sexual relations are justified so long as both partners simply understand and respect each other's motives. In any case, young people today openly and casually discuss all kinds of behavior and all shades of opinion without occasioning the shock they would have in an earlier time (at least not among their contemporaries).

One reason young people are tolerant of each other's sexual behavior—whether far-out or conservative—is that, under the post-youth-revolution code generally accepted, they do not presume to judge what is right for one another. They believe in the right of each individual to make up his or her own mind on virtually all matters, including sex. This reinforces the trend toward openness because, when there is no threat of peer-group disapproval, young people feel much less pressure to conceal what they do. (As recently as the early 1960s, young people frequently acknowledged that they felt guilty about premarital sex, even when, intellectually, they approved of it; by 1970, surveys of sexual attitudes among young people indicated that guilt over sex was an infrequent phenomenon.) Decisions concerning the relationships which justify physical intimacy to various extents, the ways in which sexual tensions may be handled or released, and the obligations or lack of obligations in any relationship between a man and a woman—all are regarded as prerogatives of the individual and not of society.

This tolerance for diversity in life styles extends in the case of many young people to an acceptance, at least in principle, of variations including communal marriages and homosexuality. And even those who support traditional moral codes for themselves tend to argue that the choice of behavior belongs to the individual.

AN EVALUATION OF THE NEW ATTITUDES

In the foregoing, I have attempted to offer a nonjudgmental report of the way things are today with young people and sex. Let me now offer some evaluative observations.

Whether the current scene as outlined above is preferable to that of an earlier day when standards were "high" and violations less visible obviously is debatable. For the college student there are both advantages to the new outlook and problems which are raised or made more acute by it. Knotty questions exist as to the meaning of new developments in individual and social morality, and of the impact of these on traditional institutions, including marriage and the family.

It is certainly true that the new freedom and openness about sex means that an individual growing up today can confront sexuality as essentially good, desirable, and welcome. A great variety of adult role models is available in addition to the parental ones, and the general acceptance of diversity in sexual expression helps the young person who, for some reason, usually originating in childhood, has trouble achieving adult sexuality to make an acceptable adjustment. The lonely, the emotionally retarded, the unsure, the ambivalent, all find it easier to establish sexual relationships than they did in an earlier day when only the "normal" was permissible or admissible. Those whose lives might have been marred by reticence, inhibition, or perhaps even deviance find it easier to establish something closer to a fully satisfactory sexual relationship.

The new freedom does not, however, solve all the sexual problems of mankind. Some may be partly eradicated or partly concealed by the new values, but others have sprung up, particularly for adolescents and people of college age, even though many have relationships that are mature and fulfilling.

Probably the most fundamental problem stemming from the increase in sexual activity among the young is that, while they may be sexually mature, many people of college age are still emotionally and socially far from mature. Competence in sexual technique, even with a variety of partners, does not necessarily carry with it the ability to form a strong, enduring relationship. Today's sexual freedom makes it easier than ever before for young people to give the impression of being quite adult and sexually sophisticated, while being in fact too immature to invest a relationship with the emotional and creative meaning essential to its ultimate fulfillment.

The new sexual freedom may produce other undesirable consequences:

Sex may be viewed by one or other of the individuals involved as the solution to all problems. Example: A girl of 17 realizes that she has been unable to have a close relationship with another human being. She initiates a sexual relationship with a boy (who himself genuinely intends to be close to her) only to find that she cannot be close to him. While it can truthfully be said that a sexual relationship does sometimes help assuage suffering or even modify symptoms, it is useless as a cure for serious emotional problems and can actually exacerbate them.

Furthermore, when, as is sometimes the case, sex is used by an immature partner simply to externalize irrational feelings—sadistic, masochistic, exploitative, or whatever—a potentially good personal relationship may be irreparably damaged. Some young people rationalize or romanticize their desires so strongly that they persuade themselves that they "love" the other person, when in fact they lack the ability—indeed even the interest—to understand the partner's feelings or to bring him any commitment on which a strong relationship might be built. Others with greater distortions of motivation may choose superficial heterosexual relationships merely to avoid the possibility of succumbing to homosexual urges of which they may be unaware or barely aware. The person searching for a successful relationship under these circumstances may cause serious hurts to others without doing him or herself much good.

When a relationship is based on problems like these—when the sexual dimension represents merely an attempt to dominate, or to express hostility, or even to control one's feelings of emptiness, dependency, or anxiety—there is little potential for growth in the individual or in the relationship, however free and natural the sex may seem to be.

PRESSURES FOR INVOLVEMENTS

Sexual relationships may be precipitated by peer social pressure before the individuals are ready for them psychologically or emotionally. The greatly increased availability, and acceptability, of sexual stimuli in the media (from the nudity of *Playboy* to hard-core pornography), the boasting of sexual activity even when it has not happened (one tradition that is yielding reluctantly to the times), and the new emphasis on sex as the natural concomitant of a warm relationship—all of these combine to push young people into sexual involvements which some do not really want and are not ready for. In an earlier era, young people who genuinely wanted a sexual relationship were required by "official" attitude to postpone it or keep it clandestine and feel guilty, but today they may be rushed by the climate of the times into a relationship highly unsatisfactory to one partner or the other, sometimes with even more unsatisfactory aftereffects.

CONFLICTING PERCEPTIONS OF PERSONAL COMMITMENT

Another problem—one not necessarily caused by the sexual factor, but often accentuated by it—is difficulty in arriving at a mutual agreement as to the degree of commitment involved in a relationship. Despite the generally high level of communication between men and women today, the easy attainment of a sexual relationship can lead to misunderstandings of one's partner's true feelings. To one who believes that sexual involvement still represents total commitment, a relatively normal amount of human fickleness in the partner can be devastating. A young man came to a University Health Service for help in dealing with the despair he felt when "his" girl, with whom he had had a sexual relationship for six months, started sleeping with his best friend. "He says he loves her, but he doesn't really know her very well," the young man said. "There are no standards any more."

Equally upsetting can be the discovery that one's partner has become distracted or sidetracked from the original commitment and can no longer maintain it to the same intense degree. A girl came to the Health Service's office after attempting suicide because the boy with whom she had had a sexual relationship for eight months had decided that he needed to take several years of field study as a geologist and could no longer maintain an ongoing, intense commitment (though he had nothing against the girl and would have continued the relationship "as was" until he had to leave). There have always been such cases—millions of them—wherein two youthful partners did not perceive their relationship in the same way. But today in many cases the fact that the two are having sex together can deepen the emotional attachment on one side or the other and cause a break-up to be more traumatic. Indeed, the effects on an immature personality can be very damaging.

If young people are to handle such problems successfully, probably the most important quality they will need might simply be called personal strength. For, if a stable relationship has developed and includes sex, each partner must already have acquired some capacity to manage his or her own private, emotional-psychological life; that is to say, both must have demonstrated a measurable amount of maturity. And the kind of maturity to which I refer does not come automatically with entrance into a sexual relationship.

THE COMPLEXITIES OF INTIMACY

Perhaps the biggest challenge in adolescence is learning to deal with intimacy. While the complexities of intimacy are not necessarily sexual, they may be made more acute and pressing because of the existence of a sexual involvement. As children, our intimacy with adults is in the nature of a one-way street, since the adult knows much more about the personal, intimate life of the child than the child does about the activities of the adult. Adolescents, however, begin to share highly personal thoughts, feelings, and finally experiences with one another. They seek that most intimate kind of relationship, a continuing and loving one; and, under the influence of biological pressures, they begin to look for potential partners.

But they are inexperienced in establishing close relationships. How does one go about it? It can be hard to admit that one feels a need for acceptance when one recognizes the possibility of rejection and fears it.

Some conscientious young people who are just in the process of learning to live with their perhaps newly discovered capacities for hostility and destruction may fear that intimacy will bring with it the temptation to hurt someone—to exploit someone for prestige or for financial or psychological reward without rendering any return—without helping their own growth and development. Others may fear that all or some of these damaging things will be done to them. Still others will enter into intimate relationships without the slightest awareness of the injury they may do to others or that others may do to them.

LEARNING THE ART OF SHARING

The kind of personal strength or maturity needed to maintain an intimate relationship successfully includes the ability to subordinate the self to the relationship even when it involves some self-sacrifice, the capacity to tolerate at least short periods of frustration (sexual and otherwise), and the willingness to work closely with a partner on a variety of practical and psychological tasks. If the boy is sick in the college infirmary, is the girl's first thought to visit him or to find someone else to go out with? If the girl is preoccupied with writing a term paper, does the boy act supportively or get turned off? If one person is touchy because of some special pressure, such as pre-exam or premenstrual tension, does the other understand or get mad and threaten to break the relationship? When he is committed to acting in a play in which she has no part, will she pitch in and work too? Such small decisions are, after all, the stuff of which meaningful relationships are made.

Clearly, older people cannot assess the new difficulties young people face in growing up today—difficulties caused by the greater sexual freedom they have asked for and we have given them—without asking: "What can we do to help them solve their new problems?"

American institutions of higher education have traditionally felt an obligation to respond to a variety of needs in the students' lives beyond the purely intellectual ones. The emphasis today, of course, is no longer on controlling the way students behave and develop during their college years but rather on providing opportunities for personal growth and for self-realization. The need for assistance in career planning, for example, has long been recognized and is handled on different campuses by various career and counseling services designed to help students think practically and effectively about the steps necessary to make the best use of their training and abilities.

COLLEGES LEND A HAND

Colleges and universities throughout the country are now similarly recognizing their obligation to assist students in facing the issues and problems inherent in human sexuality. Man's sexual nature is one of the central facts of his existence, and it affects and is affected by all the aspects of college life: academic, extracurricular, and social. The open recognition of this fact, combined with the changing sexual mores and especially the changes in the status of women, particularly in newly coeducational institutions, has led various colleges and universities to develop new types of programs in sex education and sex counseling.

There is little in such programs—or in the people making use of them—that resembles the occasional "marriage course" of the ancient '50s and '60s. Sex education itself has become vastly more technical, owing largely to increased knowledge resulting from research by specialists such as Masters and Johnson, but owing also to increased openness and acceptance of sexual topics. With so many more students becoming sexually active, the seeking of help for sexual dysfunction or personal incompatibility has become more acceptable and more natural. And the prescribing by college physicians of contraceptives—which is now being done in at least half of American university health services, as compared to only 20 per cent in 1965—has become recognized as a socially necessary and morally valid means of preventing pregnancies for which the couples are unprepared.

Here are some of the questions which are likely to be asked in such programs; I believe they represent matters that today's students—particularly those involved in or contemplating sexual relationships—need to concern themselves with:

What are some of the qualities which a warm, lasting relationship calls for, and how does one acquire or develop them?

How is a mutual sense of human dignity, actual and potential, best preserved in a continuing relationship?

How does one define an ideal relationship with a partner?

Does such a relationship involve fidelity? Continuity?

What does either partner see as crucial milestones on a possible journey to a lasting relationship?

How many of these milestones have to do with physical relations, up to and including sexual intercourse?

What happens when the partners decide to opt for a lasting relationship (marriage, or their idea of its equivalent)?

Is the individual's respect for himself or his partner increased or diminished by a sexual relationship or the lack of it, once the above decision is made?

Will it be easier or harder to create an ideal relationship later on if one has had previous sexual experience?

Will a relationship be stronger and more lasting if the individuals have their first sexual experience together?

How important is it to make public announcement of an engagement, or to have a legal marriage ceremony?

CANDID BUT LESS CASUAL

Many older conservative people, I know, are worried that the new sexual attitudes and behavior of youth are actually undermining not only the institution of marriage but also the young people's ability to make and sustain long-term, loving relationships. The truth is, of course, that attitudes toward marriage have been changing for some time, and not just among young people. If my own observations are to be trusted—and no one's are, completely, because no one sees more than the tips of numerous icebergs—many young people today are approaching the whole problem of male-female relationships in a much more serious, thoughtful, respectful way than did earlier generations. They may be more candid about sex, but they are less casual about the complexities and significance of good human relationships, including old-fashioned marriage.

Many college couples who have been sharing room and bed go on to a formal wedding and their chances for having a lasting, committed relationship are as good as any in previous generations. And there are many couples who refrain from sex before marriage—including some who do not believe in marriage in the traditional sense.

It is impossible to work with the new breed of young people, and to hear the questions they ask, without experiencing a feeling of optimism that from their honesty, their hatred of hypocrisy, and their probing determination to see life as it is, much good is coming.

1. You and two of your classmates have volunteered to participate in a senior high school class discussion on sexuality. The coordinator of the program is a physician who has for several years been active in the local University Health Service. He contacts you and asks you to let him know which aspects of the discussion you wish to present. (He will begin the program by comparing present trends in sexuality to those of former years. He wants to be sure that the discussion will bring out individual accountability.) State your choice of topics.

2. Inasmuch as you and your classmates are only two years older than the senior high school class, you may expect some candid, relevant questions directed to you. Name some of these forseeable queries.

3. Assume you have an 18-year-old son who went to college six months ago. He writes you that he has a girlfriend whom he wishes to bring home during semester vacations. He informs you that no special preparations need be made because his girlfriend will share his room. What is your reaction?

4. If the foregoing situation (#3) applied to your daughter, would your reaction be the same? Substantiate your answer.

5. In most communes, adults other than the natural parents interact rather closely with the children. Venture into some predictions about effects the communal life-style may have on children's outlook on sex and family life when they grow up to be teenagers and young adults.

Growth of the Embryo and Fetus

FERTILIZATION; SEX DETERMINATION

1. The two sex cells essential for fertilization are the __Spumatazoa__ and the __ova__.

2. Normally, the number of chromosomes in each human cell is __46__.

3. In the male and female reproductive cells (or sex cells) the number of chromosomes is __23__.

4. Explain why it is essential for the ovum and sperm to have this specific number of chromosomes.

5. The male carries two types of sex chromosomes, the __X__ chromosome and the __Y__ chromosome.

6. The sex chromosomes of the female are given the letters __XX__.

7. Briefly state which of the two parents determines the sex of the offspring and why.

male

8. Mrs. Dorothy Bing, four months pregnant, asks you if the sex of her baby is already determined. Answer her, and tell her at what time the sex of her child is determined.

firtilization

9. Draw a diagram to show Mrs. Bing what produces a boy or a girl.

10. In which structure of the female reproductive tract does fertilization usually occur? fallopian tubes

11. Describe the activity of the fertilized ovum until the time of implantation.

3 days in fallopian tubes

4 days in uterus before implanting

12. During the first two months the fertilized ovum is called embryo, and from the third month on, fetus.

13. Soon after implantation, the embryonic mass differentiates into three distinct layers of cells. These layers, from which all organs and tissues evolve, are called:

(a) entodurm

(b) mesodurm

(c) ectodurm

14. List structures derived from the germ cell layer you named under

(a) glands secreting into digestive tract

(b) muscles, bones

(c) nervous system

PLACENTA; UMBILICAL CORD

The yolk sac and chorionic villi initially provide the services for the embryo which later on are taken over by the placenta.

15. What are some of these functions of the placenta?

fetal nourishment
oxygen exchange

16. The structure connecting the placenta and the fetus is the umbilical cord.

17. It contains 3 blood vessels.

18. Contrary to the usual pattern, the two arteries carry venous blood and the vein oxygenated blood.

19. On the diagram label the circulatory vessels of the umbilical cord; indicate venous blood in blue and oxygenated blood in red. Indicate direction of blood flow (Figure 7).

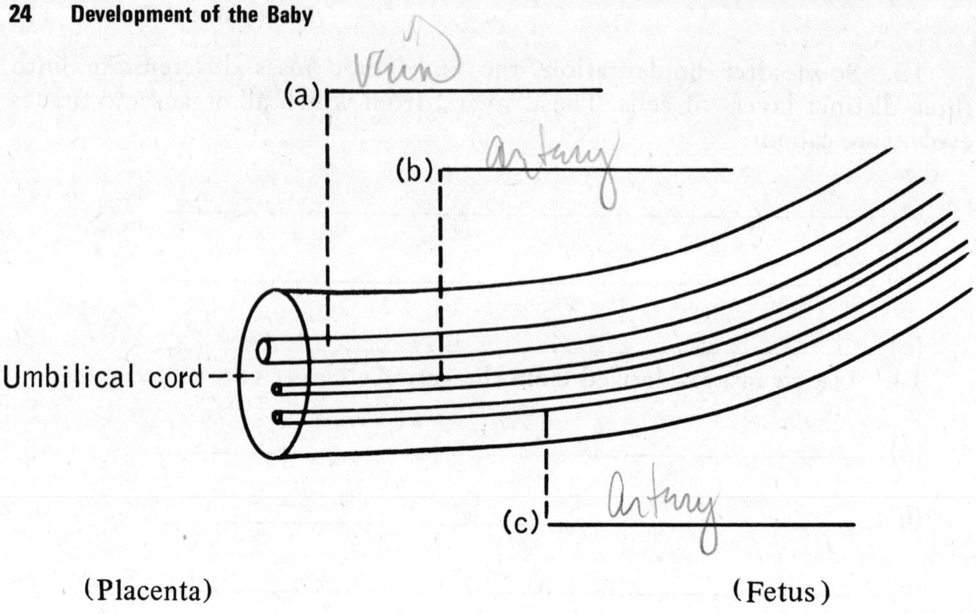

Figure 7.

FETAL CIRCULATION

In addition to the umbilical arteries and the umbilical vein there are three by-passes in the fetal circulation that are absent in the independently existing human body, in which the lungs and liver are fully functioning.

20. List the three by-passes found in the fetal circulation.

(a) ____

(b) ____

(c) ____

21. Name the two fetal by-passes that exist because the fetal lungs are not used for respiratory exchange.

(a) ______________________ which connects the ________________

with the ______________________.

(b) ______________________ which connects the ________________

with the ______________________.

22. Name the by-pass that exists because the fetal liver is not used for exchange of waste material. ______________________. It connects the ________________ with the ________________.

23. For each by-pass give the reason that makes it important that it close following birth.

(a) ____

____

(b) ____

____

(c) ____

____

24. The blackened and striated portions of the diagram indicate fetal structures that are obliterated following birth. Label them (Figure 8).

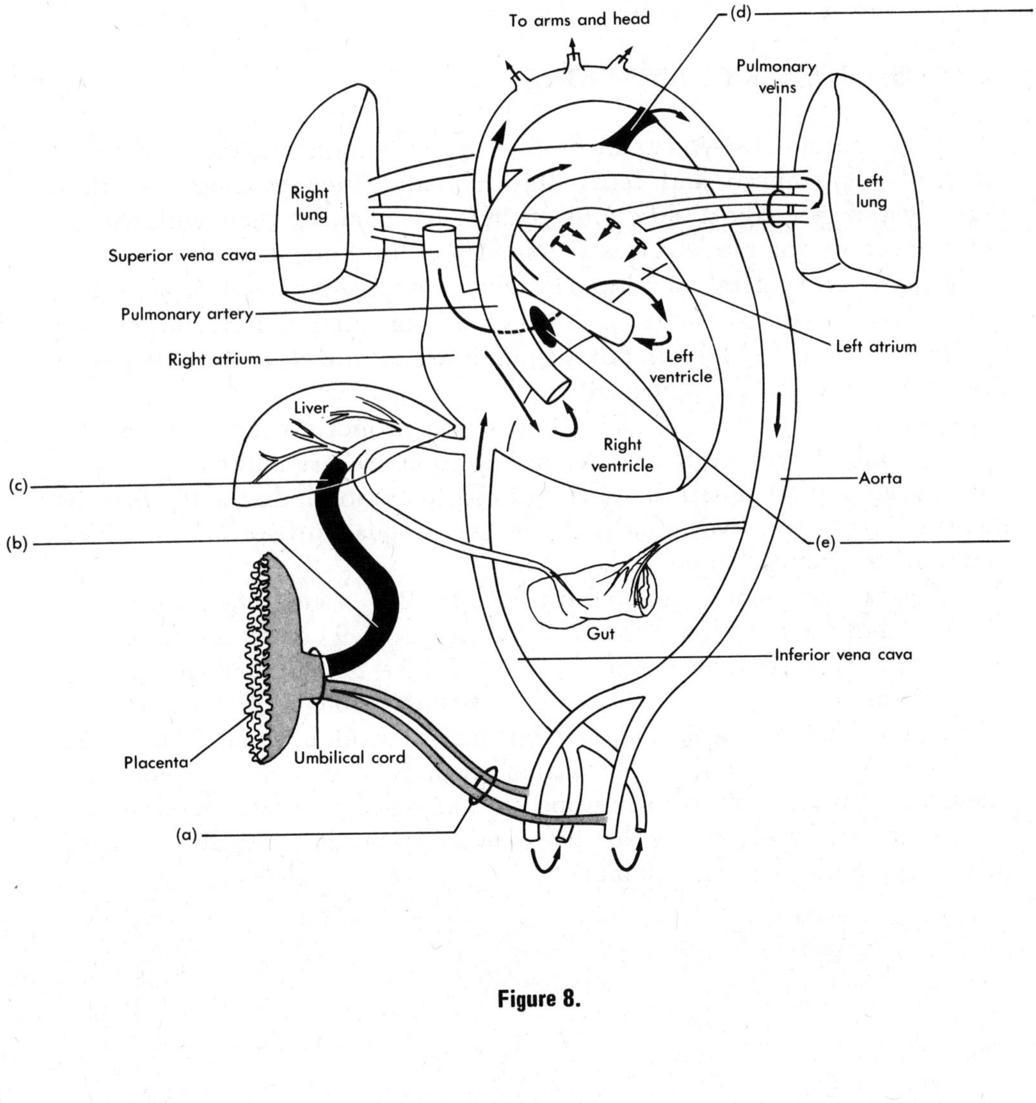

Figure 8.

FETAL MEMBRANES

25. The placenta and the fetus are surrounded by a pair of membranes. The outer membrane is called chorion ; the inner membrane is called amnion .

26. Collectively we call these membranes the ________________.

27. The sac formed by the membranes contains a slightly opaque fluid known as amniotic fluid .

28. What are some of the functions of the fluid?

29. At the end of pregnancy, how much fluid is usually found within the fetal membranes? ________________

GROWTH OF EMBRYO AND FETUS

It is important for you to be familiar with the month to month development of the embryo and fetus. Rather than trying to memorize these monthly changes, take a close look at them and compare them with changes experienced by the mother. It is a good idea to use some illustrative material showing monthly fetal development when explaining fetal growth to a mother. Such material is put out by several companies manufacturing baby foods. The book *"A Baby Is Born,"* published by the New York Maternity Center Association, is also helpful.

Remember that the rate of fetal growth is proportionally more rapid in the early months of pregnancy. According to Haase's rule, the length of the fetus in centimeters equals the square of the lunar month during the first five months. In the last five months the length is equal to five times the lunar month of pregnancy. Thus

At end of the second lunar month, $2 \times 2 = 4$ cm. fetal length
At end of the third lunar month, $3 \times 3 = 9$ cm. fetal length
At end of the sixth lunar month, $6 \times 5 = 30$ cm. fetal length
At term, $10 \times 5 = 50$ cm. fetal length

Mrs. Barbara Young is two and one-half months pregnant. This is her first baby. When you talk to her during her prenatal visit she asks you a few questions. Answer each of them using your knowledge of fetal development.

30. "You know, I have hardly gained any weight yet; do you think there is something wrong with me?"

31. "When will I be able to feel my baby move? My neighbor had her baby last month and her doctor let her listen to the baby's heart. When could I listen to mine?"

32. "Does this mean [referring to your answer to question 31] that it takes until then for my baby's heart to be formed?"

33. "Is it true that the baby swallows the fluid in which he floats?"

yes

34. "In my family most of the babies are born prematurely. Can you tell me approximately how much difference there is in the weight and length of babies born during the eighth month compared to those born at the end of the ninth month?"

MULTIPLE BIRTH

35. Define multiple birth.

36. Fraternal twins are the result of two ova, two sperm
____.

37. Identical twins are the result of one ova, one sperm
____.

38. Indicate below the difference, if any, in the structures listed.

	Identical Twins	*Fraternal Twins*
Sex		
Placenta		
Amnion		
Chorion		

39. Is there one or are there two bags of waters in twin pregnancies?

_______________ State the underlying reason for your answer.

40. In which race do twins occur most frequently, and in which least often?

41. How does multiple pregnancy tend to affect overall pregnancy?

Antepartal Care

SIGNS AND SYMPTOMS OF PREGNANCY

1. Indicate which of the following signs are positive and which are presumptive or probable for pregnancy by checking the appropriate box.

	Presumptive and Probable Signs	*Positive Sign*
(a) Frequent urination	☐	☐
(b) Morning sickness	☐	☐
(c) Palpation of the fetus	☐	☑
(d) Positive biological pregnancy test	☐	☑
(e) Softening of the cervix	☐	☐
(f) Hearing and counting the fetal heart sounds	☐	☑
(g) Cessation of menstruation	☐	☐
(h) Quickening	☐	☐
(i) Outline of fetus visible by x-ray	☐	☑
(j) Enlarged uterus	☐	☐

ANTEPARTAL VISITS

2. Discuss the advantages for mother and child of early prenatal supervision.

3. List reasons which may make it unattractive for clinic patients to seek antepartal guidance.

4. What remedial measures could be used to correct the reasons you listed?

5. You are going to work for the next six months in the large OB outpatient department of your hospital. List below the members of the health team with whom you may expect to come in contact.

6. The basic furniture and equipment which you will find in each examining room include:

Furniture	*Equipment*

7. List five items included in a thorough history taken at the first antepartal visit.

(a)

(b)

(c)

(d)

(e)

8. State the reason for performing each of the following laboratory tests during the antepartal period:

Test	*Reason*
(a) Urinalysis	
(b) Hemoglobin determination	
(c) Hematocrit determination	
(d) Serology test for syphilis	
(e) Sickle cell test	
(f) Determination of RH factor	
(g) Determination of blood group	
(h) Rubella immunity test	
(i) Papanicolaou smear	
(j) Chest x-ray	

9. While you are weighing Mrs. Anne Smith she asks you what will be done during her first antepartal visit. Write down your reply.

10. The EDC is most commonly figured out by ___Nagulas___ rule. It consists of taking the ___first___ day of the last menstrual period of the patient, adding ___7 days___ and subtracting ___3 mos.___, and then adding one year.

11. Mrs. Smith tells you that her last menstrual period started on May 5. You in turn inform her that her due date will be on ___Jubruay 12___.

12. The usual length of pregnancy, expressed in the following units, is:

(a) ___280___ days

(b) ___9___ calendar months and one week

(c) ___40___ weeks

(d) ___10___ lunar months

13. Check the following statements which apply to accepted antepartal care:

☐ (a) Regular checkups are essential to good antepartal care.

☐ (b) The patient's blood pressure, weight, and urine are checked at each visit.

☐ (c) X-ray pelvimetry is done routinely on all patients.

☐ (d) Monthly antepartal visits are the usual pattern for the first seven months.

☐ (e) Listening to the fetal heart tones during the second half of pregnancy is part of the antepartal checkup.

☐ (f) Blood samples for Hg and Ht determination are taken at each visit.

☐ (g) Patients should be seen bi-weekly and weekly during the last months of pregnancy.

14. The desired weight gain of a pregnant woman should be between ___ and ______ pounds.

15. Name the structures and factors which contribute to this weight gain.

INSTRUCTIONS TO THE PATIENT

Early in pregnancy the mother is given advice on various physical aspects of care which will enhance her well-being. Indicate the advice and underlying reason which you will give mothers on the following topics:

Topics	*Advice and Reason*
16. Care of teeth	
17. Clothes	
18. Exercise	
19. Relaxation–rest periods	
20. Daily bathing	
21. Care of breasts	

22. Bowel habits

23. Employment

24. Travel

25. Recreation–diversion

26. Smoking

27. Marital relations

28. Drugs

NUTRITION

In prenatal clinics, studies have shown a definite relationship between the diet of the mother and the health of the newborn infant. Mothers want to give their babies the best possible start in life. This can be the motivating factor in drawing special attention to eating habits during pregnancy.

Eating habits become especially important when we consider that the future health of mankind depends, to a very large degree, on nutritional foundations laid down during prenatal life. Nutrition in pregnancy is an issue whose time has come.

The physician or nutritionist usually provides the expectant mother with a food guide for this important period. Frequently the nurse is requested to interpret this food guide for the mother. Unless the circumstances are unusual, the mother-to-be may follow her regular diet, adding extra milk, meat, and other protein-rich foods, and more vegetables and fruits for vitamins A and C.

Half of the infant's weight, protein, and bone minerals is put on during the last eight weeks of intra-uterine life. Therefore, during the last trimester the mother's requirements are greater, percentage-wise for protein, minerals, and vitamins than for calories.

The diet should also be high in iron. The fetus stores iron for future needs. If the mother's diet is rich in iron, the infant will be born with a sufficient iron reserve to last through the months when his diet will be chiefly milk (which is low in iron). Important sources of iron are liver, other meats and eggs, dried beans and peas, green leafy vegetables, prunes, raisins, dried apricots, enriched or whole grain bread, and cereal.

It is usually recommended that the pregnant woman maintain a diet of 1800 to 2500 calories per day. In normal pregnancies, an increase in caloric intake of approximately 10 per cent is needed to permit the necessary adjustments in maternal physiology and to provide for fetal development. Every pregnant woman should receive supplemental ferrous iron, 30 to 60 mg. daily, during the second and third trimesters and through lactation, or, for the mother who does not breast feed, for two or three months postpartum. In addition, folic acid (200 to 400 μg daily) should probably be supplemented as prophylaxis against megaloblastic anemia.

Expectant and nursing mothers are usually cautioned to go light on sweets, fried foods, rich desserts, fats, gravies, and other high caloric foods during this period, to avoid gaining excess weight.

29. Mrs. Quinn, a primigravida, is 4 months pregnant. She is 22 years old and weighs 124 pounds, a normal weight for her medium-frame build. Her physician has sent her to attend a discussion on "diet during pregnancy" given by the nutritionist. After attending the discussion Mrs. Quinn returns to await her turn for her antepartal checkup. When you usher Mrs. Quinn to the examining room, you ask her how she liked the nutrition discussion. From her answer you conclude that she is not quite sure whether her diet provides enough milk for the calcium and the 80 grams of protein the nutritionist recommended. So you ask her to write down what she ate yesterday for breakfast, lunch, and dinner.

Mrs. Quinn's menu:

Breakfast	*Lunch*	*Dinner*
Coffee, sugar, cream 2 slices toast, butter and jelly Cornflakes, ½ cup ½ cup milk on cereal	Hot dog with bun Coffee, sugar, cream 1 banana	¼ Chicken French fries ½ cup Apple Sauce 1 piece Cherry Pie 8 oz. Coke

With the aid of Figure 9, show Mrs. Quinn how she can upgrade yesterday's menu.

30. Dr. Rigg asks you to help Mrs. Taylor, five months pregnant, work out a sample menu for a 2000 to 2200 calorie diet. Use Table 1 to help you in your selections, which you base on Mrs. Taylor's food preferences (fish, poultry, cereal, potatoes, and fruit). Point out substitutions that she could use. Tell her that she can use the same menues for her husband but serve him bigger portions.

Sample Menu

Breakfast–Calories		*Lunch–Calories*		*Dinner–Calories*	

Total Calories:

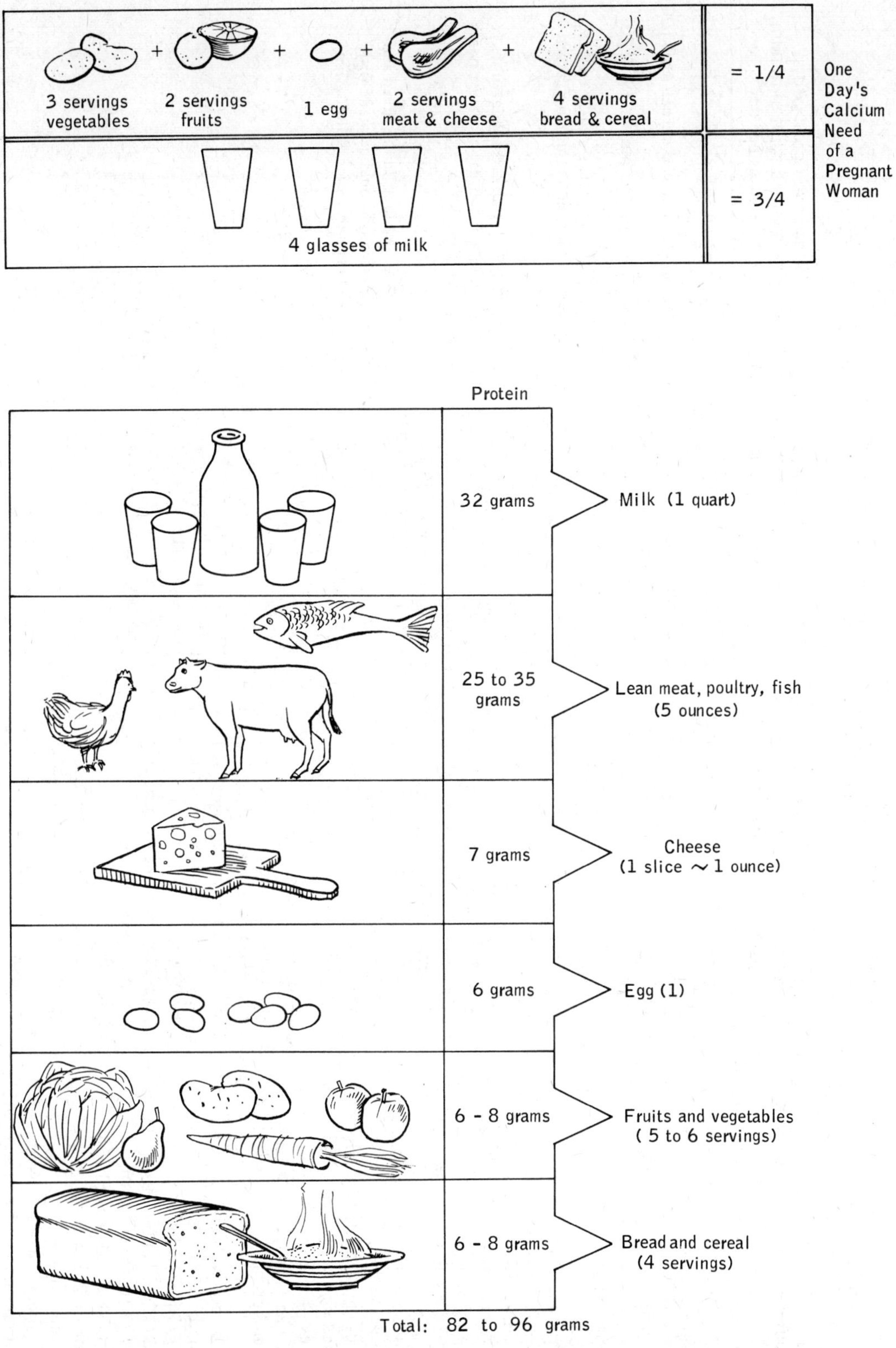

Figure 9. One Day's Protein and Calcium Needs of a Pregnant Woman

Table 1. Suggested Servings of the Four Basic Food Groups (Calories in parentheses)

Meat Group Recommended adult minimum: 4 oz. per day	Fruit and Vegetable Group Recommended adult minimum: 4 servings per day[1]	Milk Group Recommended adult minimum: 2 servings per day[2]	Bread and Cereal Group Recommended adult minimum: 4 servings per day[3]
2 to 3 oz. fish or shellfish, not counting bones or shells: 6 sardines (115) fresh or frozen fillets (avg. serving, lean, 120) ⅓ cup canned tuna or salmon (140) 4 fish sticks (160) ½ cup cooked crabmeat or lobster (180) 4 large or 9 small clams (100) ¾ cup oysters (120) 12 to 18 medium shrimp (200)	1 cup raw salad (20 or less, dressing excluded)	1 cup milk: skim (90) buttermilk (90) reconstituted nonfat dry (90) low-fat (145) whole (160) reconstituted evaporated (170) cocoa or chocolate flavored (190) malted (245)	1 slice bread (65)
2 to 3 oz. poultry, not counting skin, bone, or fat: 1 small chicken leg or thigh (90) ½ small chicken breast (155) 2 slices (4 x 2¼ in.) chicken (160), turkey (160), game hen (180), or duck (200)	½ cup cooked or canned fruit: without sugar (40 avg.) with light syrup (60 avg.) with medium syrup (80 avg.) with heavy syrup (100 avg.)	1 oz. slice Swiss cheese (105)	½ to ¾ cup cooked cereal (60-100)
2 to 3 oz. cooked lean meat, not counting bone or fat: 2 slices (4 x 2¼ in.) veal (120), lamb (130), liver (130), beef (140), ham (160), or pork (175) 1 thick or 2 thin lamb chops, trimmed (140) 2 to 3 slices Canadian bacon (160) hamburger patty (3 x ½ in.) (245)	½ cup cooked vegetables: beets, carrots, onions, peas, pumpkin, squash (35 avg.) leafy greens, asparagus, broccoli, Brussels sprouts, cabbage, celery, eggplant, string beans, tomatoes (20 or less avg.) corn, lima beans, potatoes, etc. (70 avg.)	1 cup yogurt: partially skimmed (125) whole-milk (150) with sweetened fruit added (250)	1 roll, biscuit, or muffin (90-120)
	Raw fruit: 1 medium cantaloupe (30) ½ cup berries or mixed fruit (40) 10 to 12 grapes or cherries (40) ½ medium banana or grapefruit (40) 2 medium or 3 small plums (65) 2 nectarines (65) 2 figs (80) 1 medium or 2 small peaches, pears, oranges, or apples (80)	1 cup baked custard (305)	1 oz. (about 1 cup) ready-to-eat cereal (110, not counting cream and sugar)
	6 oz. unsweetened fruit juice (80)		½ to ¾ cup cooked macaroni, spaghetti, noodles, or other pasta (100-150)

[2] Servings of milk products having a low calcium content count less than full servings. For example, ½ cup ice milk (100 calories) equals ⅓ serving; ½ cup ice cream (125 calories) equals ¼ serving; ½ cup creamed cottage cheese (130 calories) equals ⅓ serving.

[3] All products in the Bread and Cereal Group should be made with whole grain or enriched flour.

2 eggs (160)

2 to 3 oz. cheese:
½ cup cottage cheese (130)
2 slices or cubes cheddar (230)

1 cup cooked dried peas, beans, or lentils (200 avg.)

⅓ cup peanuts (280)

4 tablespoons peanut butter (380)

½ cup nut meats (almonds, cashews, walnuts) (400 avg.)

4 tablespoons vegetable protein chips (150)

[1] Vitamin C-rich fruits and vegetables: citrus fruits (oranges or juice, grapefruit or juice, tangerines or juice, lemons or juice), cantaloupe, papaya, strawberries, tomatoes or juice, Brussels sprouts, broccoli. Vitamin A-rich vegetables: deep yellow (e.g. carrots), dark green (e.g. collard greens).

31. Kari Baksh is a 17-year-old Indian girl, living with her family and expecting a baby that she plans to keep without marrying. Her family has been in the United States for five years. She is three months pregnant. While talking with her about antepartal care you find out that her diet is lacking to a great extent in vital proteins such as meat and milk. She mentions that her family seldom eats fresh fruit. After she agrees to another antepartal visit this coming Friday (when her mother can accompany her), you tell her that the purpose of the second visit is to inform her mother how to adjust Kari's diet to the demands of her pregnancy without eliminating the foods the family has been accustomed to.

On Friday you meet Kari and Mrs. Baksh and point out to them that their present ethnic diet is deficient for Kari and her expected baby. Name the foods that have been found necessary for the health of both offspring and mother. Make it clear that at this time additions to the present diet are meant only for Kari. Basing your knowledge on Kari's previous information and Indian diet in general, list the foods to be added.

32. Do you consider it advisable to mention to Mrs. Baksh that Kari's calorie intake can be higher than that of other members of the family? Give the underlying reason for your decision.

33. During your interview with Mrs. Baksh you get the impression that the mother-daughter relationship is close. Mrs. Baksh tells you she is concerned about Kari being unable to complete her senior year of high school. What is your response? List the opportunities available to Kari and her mother.

WARNING SIGNALS

The patient, during one of her first antepartal visits, should be instructed, without causing undue alarm, to report warning symptoms without delay to her physician.

34. Check which of the following symptoms you would instruct the patient to report to her physician at once:

- ☐ (a) Fatigue
- ☑ (b) Vaginal bleeding
- ☑ (c) Abdominal pain
- ☐ (d) Insomnia
- ☑ (e) Swelling of hands, legs, or face, especially upon arising
- ☐ (f) Heartburn
- ☑ (g) Failure to feel the movement of the baby over a prolonged period
- ☑ (h) Frequent severe headaches
- ☑ (i) Sudden escape of fluid from vagina

DISCOMFORTS

Sometime during pregnancy most patients experience one discomfort or another. They will rely greatly on the relief measures you will be able to offer them. Record the recommendations you suggest for relief of the listed discomforts.

Discomfort	*Relief Measures*
35. Heartburn	
36. Constipation	

37. Leg cramps

38. Morning sickness

39. Swelling of legs

40. Hemorrhoids

41. Shortness of breath

42. Vaginal discharge

43. Which one of the discomforts listed usually occurs only during the first trimester? ______________________________

44. Name the discomforts which may be caused by pressure of the enlarged uterus on other structures.

Mrs. Flip, who is expecting her third baby in two months, has pronounced varicose veins which trouble her considerably. Dr. Rigg has ordered elastic stockings for her.

45. List the instructions you are giving Mrs. Flip regarding the proper wearing of elastic stockings.

46. What additional relief measures can you suggest to Mrs. Flip?

Family Adjustments and Preparing for the Coming Baby

FITTING THE BABY INTO THE FAMILY *(emotional, financial, and environmental adjustments; preparing older siblings)*

EXPECTANT PARENTS' CLASSES

PREPARATIONS FOR THE BABY

The Smiths have been married three years and have recently moved to New York City. Jim Smith is a junior advertising executive; Eva Smith works as secretary in a bank. They are expecting their first baby in seven months. At a recent party the Smiths met the Petersons and learned that they are expecting their third baby. Both Ruth and Bob Peterson spoke highly of their obstetrician, Dr. Clark, and the Smiths decided to have him also as their physician.

You meet Mrs. Smith on her first visit to Dr. Clark, for whom you work. She seems tense and you explain to her the procedures and tests. Mrs. Smith nods and says: "Oh I know about those. I am just worried about things in general."

1. What do you reply?

2. On what principle(s) did you base your reply?

3. When Mrs. Smith tells you that she will find it hard to give up her job because she likes it and is accustomed to receiving her weekly paycheck, can you discuss her concern more fully with her?

4. What inquiries on your part could help Mrs. Smith to accept her new role?

5. What positive suggestions could you offer in answer to the financial adjustment?

When Mrs. Smith is five months pregnant she tells you that she plans to work for another two months. She says the thought of giving up her job now seems easier because the expected baby seems more real. She tells you that she has read *Pregnancy and Birth* by A. F. Guttmacher, M. D., and *Nine Months to Go* by R. M. Mitchell, M. D., and that she and her husband would like to take some classes for expectant parents. You know that the hospital where Mrs. Smith will deliver offers a series of five parents' classes. You give her a schedule of the classes and tell her to register by phone. The list of classes includes: Anatomy and Physiology of the Reproductive Organs and How the Fetus Grows; Care during Pregnancy; Demonstration of Baby Bath and Layette; The Process of Labor and Delivery; and Care of the Newborn.

6. Describe the benefits which you expect the Smiths to derive from attending parents' classes.

7. What other institutions besides hospitals offer expectant parents' classes in your community?

8. What other books, in addition to the two which Mrs. Smith has read, can you suggest to her or other patients in preparation for parenthood?

When you see Mrs. Peterson during her eighth month of pregnancy, she comments: "I am worried about getting to the hospital when I go into labor. Bob takes the car to work. My mother will come one week before my due date, but what will happen if I go into labor before?"

9. Describe inquiries and suggestions that would be of help to Mrs. Peterson.

The Petersons' children are John, age 5, and Don, age 3. When you inquire if the children are looking forward to the new baby, Mrs. Peterson replies: "Well, I guess so. But Don does not want to give up his six-year crib. We bought bunkbeds and put them in John's room, because we want to move Don in with him and use Don's room for the baby."

10. How can you help Ruth Peterson solve her problem to Don's satisfaction? Are you considering, too, how John might be involved here?

11. Name the various psychophysical preparation methods which are offered in addition to expectant parents' classes.

12. What is the purpose of psychophysical preparation for labor?

13. If an expectant mother told you that she would like to participate in one of the psychophysical preparation classes but is afraid because she is not sure that she could go through labor without analgesia, how would you respond?

14. In which ways does a husband benefit by participating in Preparation for Parenthood classes?

15. Mrs. Smith asks you what articles she should buy for the baby's layette for the first six months. What do you recommend?

16. What furnishings are required for a new baby?

17. If all the items of No. 14 and No. 15 have to be newly purchased, what advice could you offer with regard to the timing of the purchases?

Black Couples

Today 50 per cent of this nation's black people have middle-class incomes. Their goals for achievement coincide with those of middle-class whites.

18. What obstetric resources (antepartal, intrapartal, and postpartal) are available to the expectant middle-class black woman?

19. What can you personally contribute in caring for middle-income blacks?

20. Marian and Dean Hills, both in their early 30s and black, are expecting their first baby in five months. They have just moved into a two-bedroom apartment in a recently integrated section of Chicago. Mrs. Hills plans to return to her position as a teacher of handicapped children two months after her baby is born; she plans to work through her seventh month of pregnancy. Both she and her husband attend the antepartal classes offered at your hospital. Following the second session they stay late to ask you several questions.

(a) What can they expect from the hospital experience in view of the fact that they are the only black couple in the class?

(b) Do you consider it unwise for Mrs. Hills to resume working instead of raising her child full-time? (Her husband works for Commonwealth Edison and they could not afford their present standard of living without her salary.) In your reply be specific in terms of options available to her and consider her educational background.

(c) The Hills wish to continue seeing their parents, who live about 100 miles south of Chicago, one weekend a month. They wonder if the baby will be ready for travel when it is six weeks old, and ask your advice on how they can spend weekends away from home in the most timesaving manner as far as bottle feeding and dressing the baby are concerned.

Adolescent Couples

21. What are some of the difficulties which adolescent parents face when the wife becomes pregnant?

22. How can adolescent parents be helped to adjust to pregnancy and parenthood?

23. Suggest ways which would enable adolescent mothers to finish high school or to get away from home for some hours during the day so that they do not feel fenced in by motherhood.

Complications of Pregnancy

BLEEDING IN EARLY PREGNANCY

Varieties of Abortion

1. Define abortion.

2. What surgical procedure is performed for incomplete abortion?

3. What is its purpose?

Mrs. Dora Cross is admitted to the Ob-Gyne floor because of vaginal bleeding that began six hours prior to admission. She is in the third month of her first pregnancy. When you help Mrs. Cross on the bedpan you notice that her Kotex pad is saturated with approximately 30 cc. of bright blood. When you assist Mrs. Cross from the bedpan, she tells you that she thinks that she expelled "something." You notice a lump of bloody tissue mixed in the urine.

4. What is your reply to Mrs. Cross while helping her put on a clean Kotex?

5. How do you dispose of the
(a) Soiled Kotex?

(b) Contents of the bedpan?

Dr. Blake, Mrs. Cross' obstetrician, comes to see her shortly after the above episode. He tells her that she aborted the fetus and that he will perform a D. and C. the next morning. He tells her not to worry. Then he adds: "It will be all right for you to get pregnant again right away, let's say following your next period."

When you return to Mrs. Cross she asks: "What is a D. and C.?"

6. What is your answer?

Then Mrs. Cross wonders out loud: "What did I do wrong? I did the laundry at the laundromat yesterday and then did some ironing. Could that have done it?"

7. Write down your response (try to impart to Mrs. Cross the knowledge we have about the causes of spontaneous or inevitable abortions).

8. Do you think it is a normal reaction for Mrs. Cross to look for something she did as the cause for the miscarriage?

9. Elaborate on the underlying reason for your answer.

10. Why, do you suppose, did Dr. Blake mention the possibility of another pregnancy in the near future at this time?

11. List the orders which you expect to find on Mrs. Cross' chart in preparation for the D. and C. tomorrow.

12. The next morning, while Mrs. Cross is in surgery, Mr. Cross asks you how long his wife will have to stay in the hospital. State the factors on which you base your answer.

13. Match the terms in the first column with the appropriate definitions in the second column:

(a) Threatened abortion	g ☐ Expulsion of the entire product of conception
(b) Therapeutic abortion	F ☐ Abortion in succeeding pregnancies
(c) Criminal abortion	A ☐ Presence of some vaginal bleeding and cramps
(d) Inevitable abortion	B ☐ Pregnancy terminated legally by a physician
(e) Missed abortion	D ☐ Persistence of bleeding and cramps; some dilatation of the cervix
(f) Habitual abortion	E ☐ Expulsion of a portion of the fetus or accessory structures
(g) Complete abortion	C ☐ Pregnancy terminated by illegal interference
(h) Incomplete abortion	H ☐ Retention of dead fetus for some time

Uterine Vacuum Aspiration. Uterine vacuum aspiration is used in some parts of the United States in place of dilation and curettage (D. and C.) for the treatment of incomplete abortion or therapeutic abortion.

To aspirate the uterus, the physician inserts one end of a sterile cannula into the uterus and attaches the opposite end to a tube that extends nearly to the bottom of a collecting bottle. Another tube near the top of the bottle leads to a vacuum pump, which draws the fetal and placental tissues out of the uterine cavity.

Physicians have found that the suction procedure is safe, technically simple, requires little or no anesthetic, and can be completed in two to four minutes. A D. and C. takes about 15 minutes. Reportedly there is less blood loss, which is attributed to the speedy technique.

Abortion Laws. The United States Supreme Court ruled in early 1973 that states may not stop women from having doctor-approved abortions within the first six months of pregnancy. The high tribunal also said that where abortions are outlawed in the final three months of pregnancy, states must permit an exception if abortion is necessary to preserve the life or health of the mother. The justices stated that a doctor's medical judgment concerning the mother's health may involve not only physical but emotional, psychological, family, and age factors as well.

The ruling struck down state laws that up to then forbade all abortions except those necessary to preserve the mother's life. In the first three months of pregnancy, states can no longer interfere at all with a woman's private right to have an abortion, if she has her doctor's approval. In the second three months, the states may regulate where an abortion is performed, who performs it, and other conditions that may affect the well-being of the mother. Once an unborn child is viable, the states may forbid abortions unless they are required to save the mother's life or health.

The Court declared:

"We need not resolve the difficult question of when life begins. When those trained in respective disciplines of medicine, philosophy and theology are unable to arrive at any concensus, the judiciary at this point in its development of man's knowledge is not in a position to speculate as to the answer.

For the state prior to approximately the end of the first trimester, the abortion decision and its affectuation must be left to the medical judgment of the pregnant woman's attending physician.

For the stage subsequent to approximately the end of the first trimester, the state, in promoting its interest in the health of the mother, may, if it chooses, regulate the abortion procedure in ways that are reasonably related to maternal health.

For the stage subsequent to viability, the state, in promoting its interests in the potentiality of human life, may, if it chooses, regulate and even proscribe abortions except where it is necessary for the preservation of the life or health of the mother.

The decision leaves the state free to place increasing restrictions on abortion as the period of pregnancy lengthens so long as those restrictions are tailored to the recognized state interests."

Since the passage of the liberalized abortion law, hospitals and clinics have set up facilities to respond to the demand for legal abortion. The Women's Liberation Groups and previous advocates of abortion-on-demand advise women where they can have an abortion without red tape (which usually entails a waiting period).

On the other side, however, groups which opposed abortion before the new ruling remain set against it. Women might, therefore, still need to travel to distant communities to have the needed procedure carried out. It is unlikely, though, that the extremely conservative groups will be able to negate the liberalized abortion law.

14. If her doctor approves, a woman may have an abortion without state interference during which time in her pregnancy?

15. What impact does the liberalized abortion law have on:

(a) An unwed and pregnant teenager

(b) A low-income-group woman in her eighth unwanted pregnancy.

16. Does the law specify where abortions must be performed during the first three months?

17. For the sake of the well-being of the mother, the states may set up regulations for the performance of abortion from which time on during pregnancy?

Ectopic Pregnancy

18. Define ectopic pregnancy.

19. In what parts of the body may an ectopic pregnancy occur?

20. What is the most common site?

fallopian tubes

21. List the symptoms of ectopic pregnancy.

22. At what period of pregnancy do these symptoms usually appear?

After the diagnosis of ectopic pregnancy is made, the treatment is always surgery: in tubal pregnancy, excision of the affected part if rupture has not yet occurred; after rupture, removal of the affected tube.

23. What significance does tubal pregnancy play in the future obstetric history of the patient?

Hydatidiform Mole

24. Describe the symptoms of hydatidiform mole.

25. What is the treatment?

After the expulsion of a mole, the patient is carefully watched for one year, and frequent hormone (Chorionic gonadotropin) pregnancy tests are made with serum or urine. A positive reaction indicates that some living chorionic tissue is left. This must be removed after the possibility of a pregnancy is ruled out, for it is known that hydatidiform mole may predispose the patient to choriocarcinoma.

BLEEDING IN THE LAST TRIMESTER OF PREGNANCY

Abruptio Placentae; Placenta Previa

26. Define abruptio placentae.

separation of placenta early

27. Define placenta previa.

bleeding due to low implantation

28. On the diagram, label the type of placenta previa indicated (Figure 10):

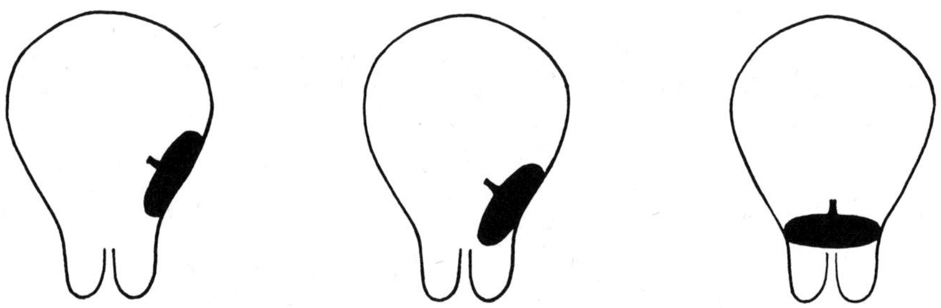

(a) ____________ (b) ____________ (c) ____________

Figure 10.

29. List two predisposing factors of placenta previa:

(a) ______________________________

(b) ______________________________

30. What is the characteristic symptom of placenta previa?

painless bleeding

31. Describe the underlying cause of this symptom.

If it is decided to deliver a patient with placenta previa vaginally, you may have to assist the physician in rupturing the patient's membranes.

32. What is the purpose of this procedure in the treatment of placenta previa?

33. What are your responsibilities in setting up for it?

34. For what types of placenta previa is cesarean section indicated?

35. In what way can you ascertain the status of the fetus of a mother diagnosed as having placenta previa?

36. What would indicate to you that the fetus was in distress?

37. Would you report to the physician a fetal heart rate:

Below 100?	Yes	☑	No	☐
Above 160?	Yes	☑	No	☐

38. State what may be indicated by a rise or fall in fetal heart tones:

contractions

39. What are some predisposing factors to abruptio placentae?

40. The bleeding of abruptio placentae is usually accompanied by what other symptom differentiating it from placenta previa?

41. If the blood escapes from the vagina in abruptio placentae, the bleeding is called ________________ .

42. If the blood is retained within the uterine cavity, it is called ______ hemorrhage.

The latter type is much more severe, but also occurs less frequently. A serious sequela to abruptio placentae is shock caused by loss of blood.

43. Indicate the effects of shock on the following:

Blood Pressure ________________________________

Pulse ________________________________

Extremities ________________________________

Oxygen supply to the brain ________________________________

44. What would you do if you diagnosed the symptoms of shock?

Treatment of abruptio placentae depends on its severity and the extent to which labor has progressed. If contractions have begun and the bleeding is only slight, labor is usually allowed to proceed normally. Rupture of the membranes so that the uterus can contract around the fetus may help to control bleeding. Rupture of the membranes also hastens labor and delivery. If labor does not proceed fairly rapidly, or if bleeding is profuse, delivery by cesarean section may be necessary to save the baby and to allow the uterine muscle to contract, thus stopping the bleeding by closing the uterine blood vessels. Replacement of blood is started before surgery is begun.

In some cases of abruptio placentae there is a failure of the blood-clotting mechanism due to a decrease in the blood fibrinogen level. To correct hypofibrinogenemia, fibrinogen is administered intravenously.

45. Indicate which of the following statements apply to abruptio placentae:

(a) All patients with abruptio placentae are delivered by cesarean section.

(b) In some cases of abruptio placentae a decrease in blood fibrinogen may occur.

(c) If labor has started and bleeding is slight, the patient may be allowed to continue labor normally.

(d) In case of profuse bleeding, or if labor does not progress fairly rapidly, cesarean section is the treatment of choice.

(e) In abruptio placentae it may be necessary to administer blood and/or fibrinogen.

46. Indicate which of the following symptoms you would check immediately after admitting a patient with abruptio placentae or placenta previa:

(a) Vital signs

(b) Amount of active bleeding

(c) Vomiting

(d) Signs indicating fetal distress

(e) Presence or absence of abdominal pain

(f) Urinary frequency

(g) Presence or absence of contractions

Mrs. Peters, eight months pregnant, is admitted to the labor and delivery suite because of vaginal bleeding. Her admission diagnosis is (a) possible placenta previa, and (b) rule out abruptio placentae. Her physician orders the following:

(a) Type and crossmatch 1000 cc. of whole blood, and have blood in delivery room before vaginal exam is carried out

(b) Prep abdomen and perineum

(c) Get legal permits signed

(d) 1000 cc. of 5% Dext./H_2O started with large intracatheter

(e) Prepare delivery room with double setup

47. Give brief explanation for each of the above orders:

(a)

(b)

(c)

(d)

(e)

While you prep Mrs. Peters you notice that she is apprehensive. She asks you: "Will my baby be all right?" (Before you started the prep, you listened to fetal heart tones and you counted 120 per minute.)

48. How will you answer Mrs. Peters?

49. What can you do to diminish Mrs. Peters' anxiety?

Mrs. Peters is delivered of a 4 lbs. 8 oz. girl by cesarean section, following a diagnosis of partial placenta previa. You are assigned to take care of Mrs. Peters in the recovery room for the three hours that remain of your eight-hour duty.

Mrs. Peters is receiving an I.V. infusion of whole blood, which is to be followed by 1000 cc. of 5% Dext./H_2O; her urinary catheter has been removed at the end of the operation; she has had spinal anesthesia and is allowed sips of water; among her orders is one for Demerol 75 mg. every 4 hrs. p.r.n.

50. List the nursing measures which you will carry out in caring for Mrs. Peters.

At 3 p.m., when it is time for you to leave, you give a report to Miss Sullivan, LPN, who is coming on duty and taking over for you.

51. List below the items which you will include in your report concerning Mrs. Peters.

COMPLICATIONS PECULIAR TO PREGNANCY

Incompetent Cervical Os

In a typical case of incompetent cervical os the cervix dilates painlessly during the fourth or fifth month of pregnancy. The membranes later rupture, labor begins, and an immature fetus is delivered. The cause of cervical incompetency is not known, but previous trauma to the cervix may be a factor. It usually does not occur in primigravidas.

52. What treatment is available to correct an incompetent os?

53. What precautionary measure is taken following correction to prevent undue pressure on the cervix?

54. While taking care of a patient who has had a modified Shirodkar operation the same morning, you are watching for signs of _______________ or _____________________.

55. If it is decided that the patient will deliver vaginally, what needs to be done at the end of the pregnancy before she goes into active labor? Why?

Hyperemesis Gravidarum

56. Define hyperemesis gravidarum.

57. What contributing factors may be responsible for it?

58. What symptoms may make hospitalization advisable?

59. State the underlying reasons for ordering parenteral fluid with added vitamins and/or minerals. (For example: 1000 cc. of 5% Dex./lactated Ringer's, with one ampule of Solu B Forte and 20 meq. of KC1 added.)

60. What is the value of prescribing:

(a) A tranquilizer or sedative ________________________

(b) An antiemetic or anticholinergic drug ____________________

61. Discuss the attitude you would use when taking care of a patient with the diagnosis of hyperemesis gravidarum. State the effect you expect from your approach.

62. When the patient is well enough to tolerate oral feedings, what types of food are usually initiated? Why?

63. Most cases of hyperemesis gravidarum respond to treatment; if not, what alternative might have to be resorted to?

Toxemia

64. Toxemia of pregnancy is a disease peculiar to pregnant women, which is called pre-eclampsia in its nonconvulsive stage and eclampsia in its convulsive stage. It almost invariably appears after the twenty-fourth week of gestation.

The American Committee on Maternal Welfare set up the following classification of toxemia:

I. *Acute toxemia of pregnancy* (onset after twenty-fourth week of gestation)
   - A. Pre-eclampsia
     1. Mild—B/P is 140/90 or more; a rise of 30 mm. or more of the systolic B/P or a rise of 15 mm. or more of the diastolic B/P; edema and proteinuria, separately or together.
     2. Severe—B/P is 160/110 or more; proteinuria of 5 gm. or more in 24 hours, equal to 3 or 4 plus on qualitative examination; oliguria, 400 or less per 24 hours; cerebral or visual disturbances; pulmonary edema or cyanosis.
   - B. Eclampsia—characterized by the same signs as pre-eclampsia with superimposed convulsions and/or coma.

II. *Chronic hypertensive (vascular) disease with pregnancy*
   - A. Without superimposed acute toxemia (no increase of hypertension or development of proteinuria).
     1. Those cases in which hypertension was definitely known to have existed before the onset of pregnancy.
     2. Cases of early hypertension discovered in pregnancy (before the twenty-fourth week of gestation and with postpartum persistence).
   - B. Chronic hypertensive vascular disease with superimposed toxemia.

III. *Unclassified toxemia* (Data insufficient to differentiate the diagnosis.)

65. Place A or B in the squares to indicate how you would categorize the descriptions given:

A. Acute hypertensive disease occurring only in pregnancy

B. Chronic hypertensive disease not peculiar to pregnancy

☐ (a) Occurs after the twenty-fourth week of pregnancy

☐ (b) Severe pre-eclampsia

☐ (c) Usually occurs before the twenty-fourth week of pregnancy

☐ (d) Mild pre-eclampsia

☐ (e) May be superimposed by acute toxemia

☐ (f) Eclampsia

Within which group of women does toxemia occur more frequently?

Mrs. Ann Davis, age 17, arrives at the physician's office and tells you that she cannot remove her wedding band because her fingers seem to have swollen. She is seven months pregnant, and on reading her chart you notice that during previous prenatal visits her blood pressure has been 110/72 to 116/74, her urine has been negative for albumin and sugar; her weight gain increased from an initial 110 lbs. to 117 lbs. on her last visit. After taking care of Mrs. Davis you enter the following findings on her chart: B/P, 142/96; weight, 128 lbs; increased striae marks on abdomen; FHT, 148; urine negative for sugar, with a trace of albumin; edema of feet and hands; complains of tiredness and constipation.

66. Are there any abnormal findings in your entry on the patient's chart? ______ If so, which ones?

67. If you consider the symptoms exhibited by Mrs. Davis, are these the initial signs of toxemia? _______ If not, what are the symptoms of toxemia?

Dr. Franklin instructs Mrs. Davis to get extra rest, to drink 2000 to 2500 cc. of fluids per day and to start on a low-salt diet. In addition, he orders Hydrodiuril, 25 mg. every 12 hours.

Before Mrs. Davis leaves the office you explain to her more explicitly why the above instructions are necessary for her well-being.

68. What do you tell her about the importance of, and how she can accomplish, the following?

(a) Extra rest

(b) Intake of 2000 to 2500 cc. of fluids

(c) Eating a low-salt diet

69. Explain to Mrs. Davis the purpose of, and the effects she can expect from, taking Hydrodiuril.

Mrs. Ann Davis returns to the office one week later. You notice her urine is negative for albumin, her weight is 122 lbs., her B/P is 126/80. Dr. Franklin tells Mrs. Davis to stay on the previously prescribed regime, but to decrease the Hydrodiuril to 25 mg./day.

70. How can you encourage Mrs. Davis to continue the instructions given her at the last visit?

When Mrs. Davis leaves you give her a written list of symptoms, and you ask her to report promptly the appearance of any of them.

71. List the symptoms you wrote down for Mrs. Davis.

72. Check which of the following symptoms are associated with severe pre-eclampsia.

☐ (a) In severe pre-eclampsia the blood pressure rises to 140/100.

☐ (b) Severe pre-eclampsia may be characterized by a weekly weight gain of 1.5 to 2 lbs.

☐ (c) Albuminuria may rise to 6 to 8 gm. per liter.

☐ (d) One of the symptoms of severe pre-eclampsia is a blood pressure of 160/110 or more.

☐ (e) The blood protein is elevated in severe pre-eclampsia.

☐ (f) A weight gain of 2 lbs. per week or more may occur.

☐ (g) Urinary output is markedly increased.

☐ (h) Severe pre-eclampsia is characterized by convulsions.

The essentials of severe pre-eclampsia treatment are rest, increased diuresis, use of vasodepressor drugs, sedation, a low-salt diet, and close watching for unfavorable symptoms and ultimate delivery. Complete recovery is not assured until after delivery of the baby.

73. State the nursing measures which you would take to ensure utmost rest.

74. Name three drugs which induce diuresis:

(a) ______________________________

(b) ______________________________

(c) ______________________________

75. Name four vasodepressors which may be used in the treatment of severe pre-eclampsia:

(a) ______________________________

(b) ______________________________

(c) ______________________________

(d) ______________________________

76. Name three sedatives which may be prescribed for treatment of severe pre-eclampsia:

(a) ______________________________

(b) ______________________________

(c) ______________________________

77. Write out a day's menu for a low-salt diet providing 80 to 100 gm. of protein (specify whether you use fresh or canned food). Refer to Figure 9, page 37.

Breakfast	*Lunch*	*Dinner*

78. List the unfavorable symptoms to look for when taking care of a patient with severe pre-eclampsia.

79. Why is delivery at the right time, either by induction or cesarean section, the ultimate goal for treatment of severe pre-eclampsia?

(a) ____________________

(b) ____________________

(c) ____________________

80. Briefly state the reasons for the nursing care of the eclamptic patient listed on the left:

Nursing Care	*Reason*
(a) Patient should not be left unattended	
(b) Offer oral fluids only to the thoroughly conscious patient	
(c) Provide a quiet environment with subdued lights	
(d) Close observation of effects of administered drugs	
(e) Observe for signs of labor	
(f) Accurate recording of intake and output	
(g) Accurate recording of blood pressure	
(h) Accurate recording of duration and character of convulsion	

81. Indicate which of the following symptoms may appear in which phase of the toxemias by checking the appropriate box or boxes:

		Mild Pre-eclampsia	*Severe Pre-eclampsia*	*Eclampsia*	*Chronic Hypertensive Disease*
(a)	Oliguria	☐	☐	☐	☐
(b)	Symptoms disappear following delivery of baby	☐	☐	☐	☐
(c)	Edema, albuminuria	☐	☐	☐	☐
(d)	Elevated blood pressure may be diagnosed in the first half of pregnancy	☐	☐	☐	☐
(e)	Occurrence of convulsions	☐	☐	☐	☐
(f)	Blood pressure of 160/110 or more	☐	☐	☐	☐
(g)	Blurred vision or spots before the eyes	☐	☐	☐	☐
(h)	A rise in blood pressure of 25/15 mm. of mercury over an established early-pregnancy level	☐	☐	☐	☐

Rh incompatibility

82. Indicate the Rh type of the expectant mother and the Rh type of the father that may give rise to Rh incompatibility:

(a) Expectant mother ______________ (b) Father ________________

83. What would happen if the couple's Rh types were reversed?

84. List in sequence the steps which occur in Rh sensitization (formation of Rh antibodies by the mother).

85. Describe the possible effects of Rh sensitization on:

(a) The first baby ______________________________

(b) The second baby ______________________________

(c) The third baby ______________________________

(d) The fourth baby ______________________________

86. Define amniocentesis.

87. What is its purpose in Rh incompatibility?

88. The pigment which causes the darkening of the amniotic fluid in Rh incompatibility is called ____________________ .

89. Intra-uterine transfusion consists of:

____ .

90. When is it indicated?

91. What is its purpose?

92. What complications may arise following an intra-uterine transfusion?

93. Match the statements of column I with the reasons given in column II which apply to intra-uterine transfusion:

I	*II*
(a) Use of type-O negative red cells	☐ Fetus able to absorb blood cells directly from its abdominal cavity
(b) Transfusion given into the fetus' abdominal cavity	☐ In Rh incompatibility, only the baby's red cells are being destroyed
(c) Accomplishment of transfusion	☐ Immune to mother's antibodies
(d) Injection of packed red blood cells instead of whole blood	☐ Corrects baby's anemia

Rh "Vaccine." A "vaccine" for Rh-negative mothers that protects babies against hemolytic disease of the newborn is now available under the trade name RhoGAM. It promises to eliminate erythroblastosis fetalis, which menaces 10 per cent of American families (kills 10,000 babies every year in the United States, and burdens another 20,000 with congenital anemia, heart failure, jaundice, or mental retardation).

A single dose of the anti-Rh globulin is adequate to prevent a susceptible mother from developing active Rh immunity. The vaccine nullifies the antigenic stimulus of the infant's Rh-positive red cells that enter the mother's circulation, especially at the time of delivery (placental separation), and prevents a primary immune response. In a subsequent pregnancy with an Rh-positive fetus, the mother will have no Rh antibody to hemolyze the fetus' Rh-positive cells.

The decision to vaccinate Rh-negative mothers rests on the answers to several questions: Is the mother's blood free of sensitization to the Rh factor? Is her baby's blood Rh-positive, and does it give negative results to a direct Coombs test? If the answers are affirmative, a sample of the mother's blood should be crossmatched with the RhoGAM solution. If there is no incompatibility, the protective injection should be given intramuscularly within 72 hours after delivery. It is necessary to follow this procedure following each delivery and also after a miscarriage involving an Rh-positive fetus.

The vaccine does not work on Rh-negative mothers who have already acquired their own permanent active antibodies by having given birth to an Rh-positive child. Nevertheless, within the next few years hemolytic disease of the newborn should become a disorder of the past, for by then all Rh-negative mothers should have been treated with RhoGAM from the first pregnancy on.

GENERAL MEDICAL DISEASES AND PREGNANCY

Rubella

94. The lay term for rubella is ______________________ .

95. Explain the importance of preventing exposure to rubella during the first three months of pregnancy.

96. What precaution should be taken following delivery when a patient has had rubella during pregnancy? What is the underlying reason?

A new laboratory test which reliably confirms immunity to rubella has now been developed. This test is so simple and dependable that a physician can determine within three hours whether a person has been previously infected with the rubella virus by showing whether she has developed protective antibodies against it.

Rubella vaccine is now routinely administered to preschool and school-age children. The purpose of this procedure is to prevent children from contracting the disease and in turn infecting women of childbearing age.

97. Discuss the value and application of the rubella immunity test.

98. What effects pertinent to childbearing result when rubella vaccine is administered to children?

Tuberculosis

99. Differentiate between the advice a woman with old, healed tuberculous lesions would get concerning becoming pregnant and a woman having active tuberculosis.

100. Check the following statements which apply to tuberculosis during pregnancy.

- ☐ (a) The treatment of the tuberculosis of an expectant mother is the same as if pregnancy were not superimposed.
- ☐ (b) Adequate rest and administration of two of the three antimicrobial drugs (streptomycin, isoniazid, and PAS) are part of the treatment.
- ☐ (c) Pregnancy is not a contraindication for surgical intervention in active tuberculosis if it is done before the third trimester.

☐ (d) Patients with tuberculosis should not be given any medication during labor.

☐ (e) The second stage of labor should be shortened by the use of forceps for delivery.

☐ (f) It is the aim of good obstetrics to provide an uncomplicated labor for the tuberculous patient to prevent exhaustion and blood loss.

☐ (g) Antimicrobial therapy during pregnancy has not been found to have an undesirable effect on the developing fetus.

☐ (h) Children born to women with active tuberculosis are separated from their mothers following delivery to prevent exposure to the infection.

Heart Disease

Mrs. Leonore Court, 24 years old, is two months pregnant. This is her first pregnancy. She attends cardiac clinic because of impaired heart valves which resulted from rheumatic fever when she was 11 years old. Mrs. Court's husband is a car mechanic who works 12 hours daily, except Monday. She tells you that her relatives are all living out of town.

After examining Mrs. Court, Dr. Yard tells her that he is satisfied with her present health, but that she should take it easy, rest a lot, follow the 2000-calorie diet he gave her (no salt to be used in preparation of food), and that he wants to see her again in two weeks.

101. How does pregnancy affect the heart?

Before Mrs. Court leaves, you talk with her about Dr. Yard's recommendations. You ask her about her daily activities and find out that she lives in a second-floor apartment.

102. What do you recommend to her about:

(a) Sleep and rest periods during the day

(b) Activities which involve climbing stairs (shopping, doing laundry, and so forth)

(c) General hygiene

(d) Diet

(e) Diversion–recreation

(f) Household activities

103. Why did Dr. Yard ask Mrs. Court to see him again in two weeks?

104. What extra observations and measures should be instituted for Mrs. Court during:

(a) Labor

(b) Delivery

(c) Postpartum

Diabetes Mellitus

You have been asked to be the panel leader of a round table discussion on "diabetes and pregnancy." Your group's presentation is to be held at the clinical meetings of the Practical Student Nurses' convention.

You assign the following topics to the participants:

Participant 1—Antepartal care of diabetic patient.

Participant 2—Complications associated with diabetes in pregnancy.

Participant 3—Delivery plans for the diabetic patient, and special nursing observations during labor and puerperium.

A day before the panel presentation you meet with your group, and each participant discusses her material. Outline your group's presentation.

105. *Participant 1*—Antepartal care of diabetic mother.
Topics and reasons

106. *Participant 2*—Complications associated with diabetes in pregnancy.
Topics and reasons

107. *Participant 3*—Delivery plans for the diabetic patient, and special nursing observations during labor and puerperium.

Topics and reasons

Syphilis

108. If an expectant mother with active syphilis is not treated, pregnancy may be terminated by:

(a)

(b)

109. Complete the following details of the treatment for syphilis:

(a) Name of drug:

(b) Dosage:

(c) Route of administration:

(d) Length of treatment:

Adequate treatment of the mother during the first 18 weeks of gestation consists of preventing infection of the fetus. Treatment after the eighteenth week of gestation consists of treatment of the infant in utero.

110. Give the underlying factors for the above statement.

111. Explain why the VDRL test of a treated patient may be positive at the time of delivery.

112. Does the statement of No. 111 mean that the baby will have congenital syphilis? ________ Give the reason for your answer.

Gonorrhea

According to statistics released by the government's Center for Disease Control in Atlanta, reported cases of gonorrhea are at the highest level in United States history and exceed by far the combined cases of all other communicable diseases. Between two million and three million persons in the United States have gonorrhea.

The infectious agent that causes gonorrhea is a bacterium, the gonococcus, Neisseria gonorrhoeae. This organism is quickly destroyed outside the body and is sufficiently specialized to require transfer between hosts via the mucous membranes of the genitals, mouth, or rectum. It cannot be transferred through breaks in the skin or through cuts; it is not transferred across the placenta. It is transmitted to the baby's eyes during birth while he is passing through the vagina. Untreated it will cause blindness by scarring and fibrosis. Because of this, all states require the eyes of newborn babies to be treated with 1 per cent silver nitrate or an antibiotic preparation.

The U.S. Food and Drug Administration has now approved a drug that can cure gonorrhea in one dose. It is called Polycillin PRB and the patient is usually cured within 48 hours. Gonorrhea patients who are sensitive to penicillin are given alternate therapy consisting of oral tetracycline in a 1.5 gm. initial dose followed by 0.5 gm. doses every six hours for a total of 9 gm.

Gonorrhea occurs most often in the 15 to 25-year-old age group. While the disease usually does not spread to the pelvic cavity during pregnancy, it does so before and following pregnancy if it is not treated. It may thus cause pelvic inflammatory disease. Once the infection reaches the tubes and ovaries, the inflammatory reaction, no matter how quickly treated, results in scarring and fibrosis that distorts the anatomy of the tubes; the ovum cannot then be transported from the ovary to the uterus. Sterility thus occurs in ever-increasing proportion among the younger generation.

The most important matter at hand is the treatment and prevention of gonorrhea. The subject has been discussed on television by Dick Cavett and the subsequent increase in visits to VD clinics and physicians was most rewarding. The young have to be approached in a manner acceptable to them and in a nonjudgmental atmosphere.

One of the most important recent recommendations of the National Commission on Venereal Disease, which has been especially active in combating the problem, is the modification of existing legislation to permit minors to obtain treatment for VD without parental consent. The interpersonal relationships between parents and children that make a child's access to good medical care in such cases so difficult need careful study. Parents must be made aware of the social aspects of this medical situation.

Increasing use of the pill and the intra-uterine device for contraception may have led to an increase in sexual intercourse, while at the same time reducing the prevalence of the contraceptive agent most useful in the prevention of VD: the condom. We in the health profession have an obligation to alert the young and sexually active to the pressing and real health dangers presented by venereal disease. They must also be made to understand that both males and females may spread the infection even when it is asymptomatic. This is an additional reason for stressing to them the importance of contact-tracing procedures.

113. Why is it important to trace and treat all the contacts of a gonorrhea patient?

114. Today's antibiotic dosage is many times that of 20 years ago. State the reason.

115. How long does it take to be infection-free after treatment for gonorrhea?

Clinical Course of Labor

EFFACEMENT AND DILATATION

1. Define labor.

2. What changes occur in the cervix during labor?

3. Define:
(a) Effacement

(b) Dilatation

4. In what units is cervical dilatation measured?

5. Full dilatation means the cervix is ______ dilated.
6. Indicate on Figure 11 what has taken place in sketches 2 and 3.

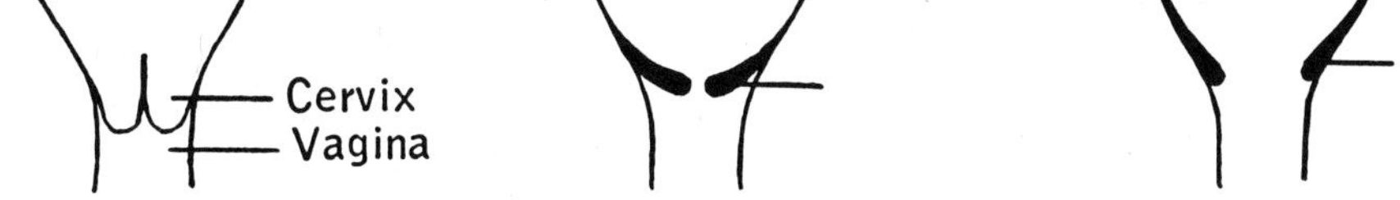

Figure 11.

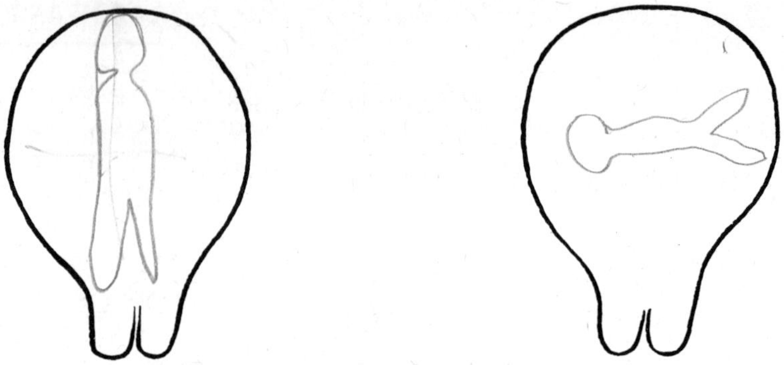

(a) Longitudinal lie (b) Transverse lie

Figure 12.

LIE OF THE FETUS

7. What is meant by the term "lie" in the phrase "lie of the fetus"?

8. Within the diagrams of the uterus (Figure 12) draw:
(a) A longitudinal lie

(b) A transverse lie

9. Explain why a transverse lie is considered a serious complication of labor.

MECHANISM OF LABOR

You find the following entries on the delivery room board:

Name	*Gr.*	*P.*	*Pres.*	*Pos.*	*Stat.*
Mrs. Alvin	v	iii	breech	RSA	−2
Mrs. Brown	i	0	ceph.	LOA	+1
Mrs. Carter	ii	0	ceph.	ROP	0
Mrs. Dunn	iii	ii	ceph.	LMA	−1

10. State the number of pregnancies, abortions, and deliveries of viable infants of:

	Pregnancies	*Abortions*	*Deliveries*
Mrs. Alvin	5	1	4
Mrs. Brown	1	0	0
Mrs. Carter	2	1	0
Mrs. Dunn	3	0	2

11. Mrs. Alvin's presentation is listed as breech. What does this indicate?

12. Write out in full the position of each patient and mark it with an "X" on the cross section of the pelvis (Figure 13).

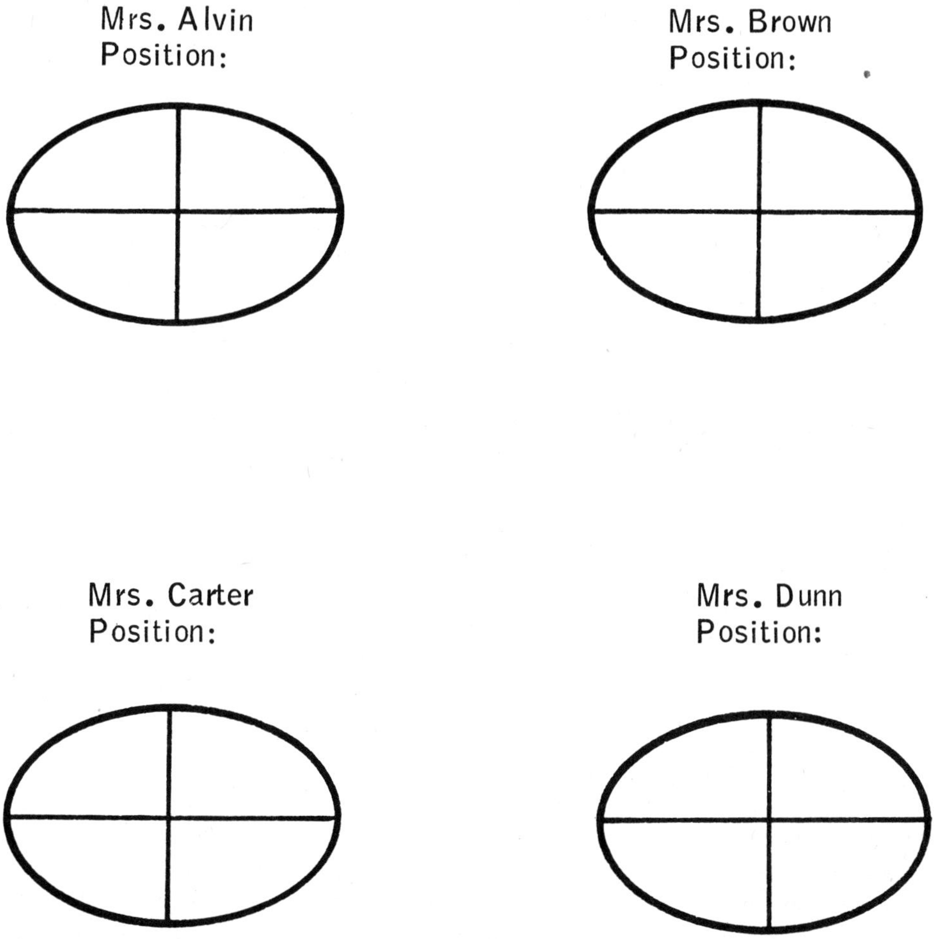

Figure 13.

13. Which of the patients has the most frequently occurring position?

14. Which patient indicates a face presentation?

15. Explain the implications of a face presentation.

16. Why does a labor in which the vertex presents in a posterior position last longer, and why is it often accompanied by back pain?

17. When the largest diameter of the presenting part has passed through the pelvic inlet, ______________ has taken place.

18. Mrs. Alvin's station is recorded as –2; Mrs. Brown's as +1. What do these entries signify, respectively?

Dr. Jackson asks you to check fetal heart tones on Mrs. Carrol. He tells you that this is her first baby and that she has been in labor 14 hours during which she has dilated only up to 3 cm. He says there is a question of cephalopelvic disproportion which he will have checked by x-ray pelvimetry.

You enter Mrs. Carrol's room and introduce yourself. You find that contractions are seven minutes apart, moderately strong, lasting 35 seconds. In order to hear the fetal heart sounds you want to ascertain fetal presentation and position. You go about this using abdominal palpation. (See Figure 14.)

Standing at the side of the bed and facing Mrs. Carrol, you gently palpate the fundus with the fingertips of both hands. You feel a soft, movable, irregular shaped object. Secondly, you press gently, but deeply with the palm or surface of your hands on each side of the abdomen outlining the fetal shape. You feel a resistant, relatively straight surface on Mrs. Carrol's left side, and irregular small parts on the right. Thirdly, you palpate the lower abdomen just above the symphysis pubis with the thumb and the fingers of one hand. You feel a hard, round object which you cannot move.

You then turn and face Mrs. Carrol's feet and again exert deep pressure downward on each side of the abdomen toward the pelvic inlet. Your left hand glides down further than your right hand over a firm surface. You cannot move the part felt.

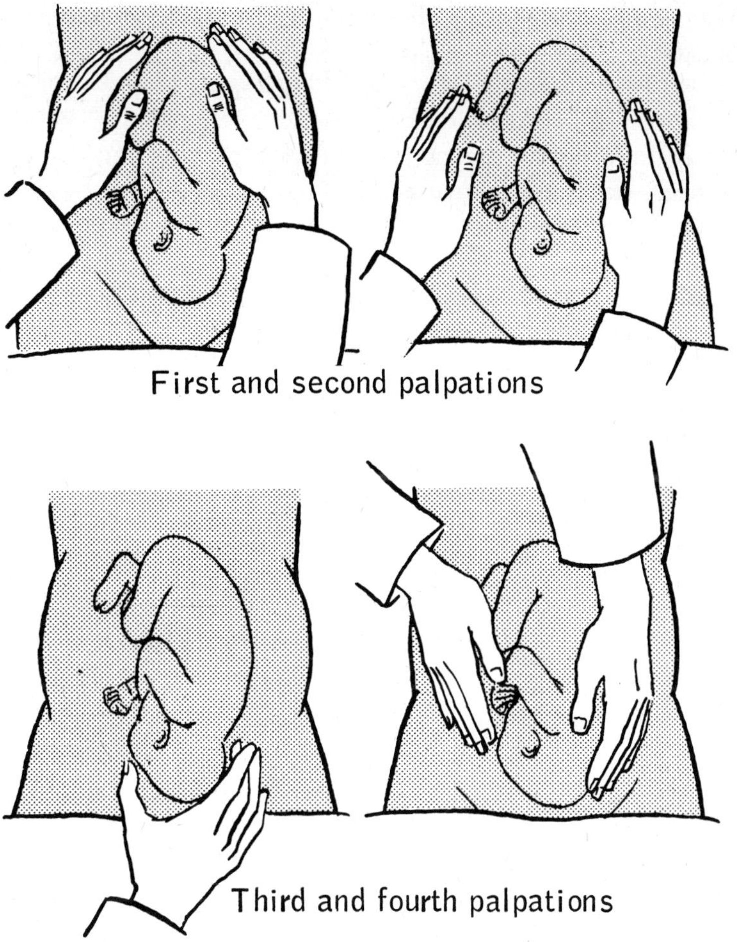

Figure 14.

19. From your findings, what seems to be the Carrol baby's:

(a) Presentation ______________________________

(b) Position ________________________________

20. Where will you place the fetoscope in order to hear the fetal heart sounds best? Give the reason underlying your action.

21. What is meant by cephalopelvic disproportion?

22. What clinical symptom described by Dr. Jackson may point toward this complication?

23. What may be the consequences of cephalopelvic disproportion if corrective treatment is not instituted?

24. State the reason why Dr. Jackson wants you to check the fetal heart tones of Mrs. Carrol.

STAGES OF LABOR

25. Which stage of labor lasts longest?

26. What is accomplished during the first stage of labor?

27. During which stage of labor is the baby being born?

28. After the birth of the baby the placenta is being expelled. This occurs during which stage of labor?

29. Match the stages of labor on the left with the description on the right:

A. The first stage

B. The second stage

C. The third stage

☐ (a) The stage of expulsion

☐ (b) Lasts from the birth of the baby until the placenta has been expelled

☐ (c) May last from 6 to 16 hours

☐ (d) The placental stage

☐ (e) Lasts from the onset of regular contractions until the cervix is completely dilated

☐ (f) May last from 15 minutes to two hours

☐ (g) The stage of dilatation

☐ (h) Lasts from full dilatation of the cervix until the baby is born

☐ (i) Usually last 5 to 20 minutes

INSTRUCTING PATIENT ABOUT LABOR AND DELIVERY

You have been seeing Mrs. Ruth Weaver several times in the clinic during her pregnancy. She is now in the seventh month of her first pregnancy and today you are performing the usual procedures of B/P, weight, and urinalysis. After you count Mrs. Weaver's fetal heart tones (152), you ask her if she would like to listen to them. She eagerly says yes, and you get the Lefoscope. After listening to her baby's heartbeat, Mrs. Weaver smiles and says: "There is so much that I would like to know about this baby. I am looking forward to his birth, but I hope I am not going to be disappointed like my girlfriend."

"What happened to your girlfriend?" you want to know.

"Oh, she had an awful time having the baby. She was in the labor-room for two days before the baby was born, and she was in so much pain that she just wanted to get it over with. She says she didn't care whether the baby lived or not. And when she saw the baby she thought he was ugly and not worth the pain she had gone through. Even now at home she is tired and says she wishes she could rest without having to get up for the baby. She does not want another baby, ever, even though her little boy is very good and cute. She says it is too awful to have them born."

"She means labor is awful?" you ask. Mrs. Weaver nods. "Do you know what goes on during labor and when the baby is born?" you continue.

"That's what I am wondering about," Mrs. Weaver replies. "I just can't quite figure it out."

You tell Mrs. Weaver that you will explain to her what happens during labor and delivery. You show her the illustrations in the birth atlas so she can see what you are describing.

30. What underlying reasons made you decide to meet Mrs. Weaver's need to have a knowledge of the physiology of labor?

31. Write down your description of labor (include a description of the uterus, the bag of waters, amniotic fluid, the purpose of labor contractions, and the length of labor). (See Figures 15 and 16.)

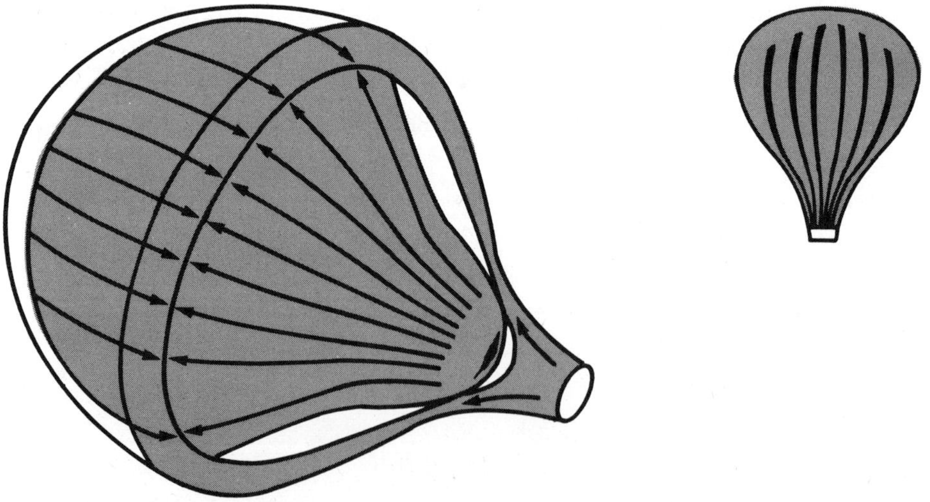

Figure 15. In these diagrams the longitudinal fibers of the uterus are shown. The arrows in the larger figure indicate the way in which the contractions both push the baby toward the outlet and at the same time efface the cervix.

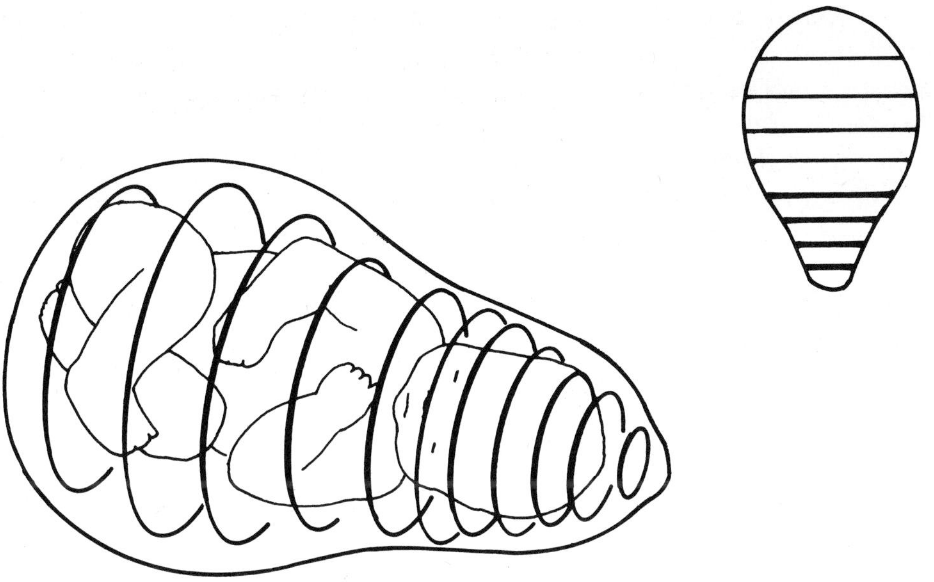

Figure 16. The two diagrams show the circular muscle fibers of the lower uterus and cervix. These fibers are the forces resisting the contractions. They must be stretched to achieve complete dilatation and permit the passage of the baby's head. Thus the expectant mother is taught to relax during a contraction to reduce the time required for this stretching.

32. Describe to Mrs. Weaver the progressive sensations of labor contractions.

33. You tell Mrs. Weaver about the breathing techniques she can use during labor and that she may be asked to push and pant. Describe each breathing technique, at what time in labor it may be used, and its purpose:

(a) Abdominal breathing

Description ________________________________

When used ________________________________

Purpose ________________________________

(b) Slow intercostal (chest) breathing

Description ________________________________

When used ________________________________

Purpose ________________________________

(c) Shallow intercostal (chest) breathing

Description ______________________________

When used ______________________________

Purpose ______________________________

(d) Pushing

Description ______________________________

When used ______________________________

Purpose ______________________________

(e) Panting

Description ______________________________

When used ______________________________

Purpose ______________________________

34. Should you mention medication during labor to Mrs. Weaver? State the reason for your answer.

35. Write down your explanation of the delivery of the baby. Include the type of anesthesia most commonly used in your hospital and the position of the mother on the delivery table; keep in mind that Mrs. Weaver is a primigravida and may need an episiotomy.

36. Mrs. Weaver asks you how she will know when she is in labor. What do you answer?

37. Based on your answer of No. 36, what do you advise Mrs. Weaver to do when she is in labor?

Before Mrs. Weaver leaves the clinic you give her a prenatal care pamphlet which has pictures and explanations of the birth process, and you tell her that you will talk again with her at her next visit.

FALSE LABOR; RUPTURE OF MEMBRANES

38. State the major differential feature between false labor and true labor.

39. What is meant by "premature rupture of the membranes"?

40. What precautions are taken after the membranes rupture?

(a) ______________________________

(b) ______________________________

41. Name two complications which may arise following rupture of the membranes.

(a) ______________________________

(b) ______________________________

42. What is the Nitrazine test? On which facts is it based?

Drugs and Anesthesia

ANALGESICS

1. State the purpose and effects of the judicious use of analgesia during labor.

2. Name the drugs and their dosages most commonly used in your hospital to achieve analgesia.

3. Discuss the rationale underlying the administration of a tranquilizer combined with a narcotic analgesic during the first stage of labor.

4. Analgesic drugs may be administered intramuscularly or intravenously during labor. You inform a patient receiving the medication intravenously that she may expect results ______________________ ; to the patient receiving medication intramuscularly, you explain that she may feel the effects ______________________ .

5. List the steps which you would take before and after administering an analgesic to a patient in active labor.

6. Discuss the reason for prescribing pain-relieving drugs only when the patient is making definite progress in labor, i.e., when the patient has reached about 4 cm. dilatation.

7. Name two narcotic antagonists.

8. Describe the action of the drugs you named in No. 7 (include when and to whom they can be administered).

9. List some adverse effects which may result from injudicious use of analgesics.

10. How can you tactfully explain the effects listed in No. 9 to a patient who is demanding repeated doses of sedatives?

11. What substitute measures would you use to make a patient who cannot receive any additional medication comfortable?

12. Why is it good practice not to administer analgesics within two hours prior to delivery?

13. When it is desirable to induce amnesia with reference to the labor contractions, the drug ____________________ is administered.

14. The drug you named in No. 13 has what additional property which makes it useful for preoperative medication?

15. Mrs. Pearl Scott's physician orders Trilene inhalations when she reaches 6 cm. dilatation. You are asked to explain the use of the inhalator, and so forth, to her. State what you included in your explanation.

16. The principle of abdominal decompression is similar to that of

_________________________ breathing, which is used during the first stage of labor.

17. Explain in what manner abdominal decompression relieves the discomfort of a contraction.

18. List the advantages of the abdominal decompressor (Birtheez suit).

GENERAL ANESTHESIA

19. Define general anesthesia.

20. Name at least five agents which may be used to administer general anesthesia.

21. List advantages and disadvantages of general anesthesia.

(a) Advantages

(b) Disadvantages

22. What precautions should be observed to prevent complications to the mother and baby from general anesthesia?

REGIONAL ANESTHESIA

23. Name the advantages of regional anesthesia to the labor patient. (See Figures 17, 18, 19, and 20.)

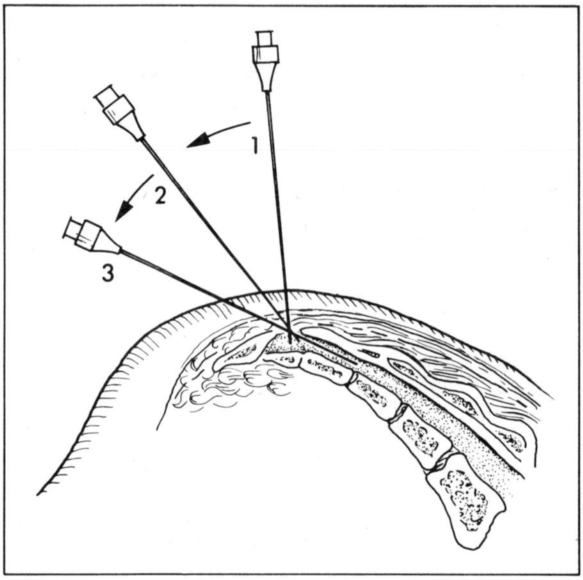

Figure 17. Insertion of Needle for Caudal Anesthesia

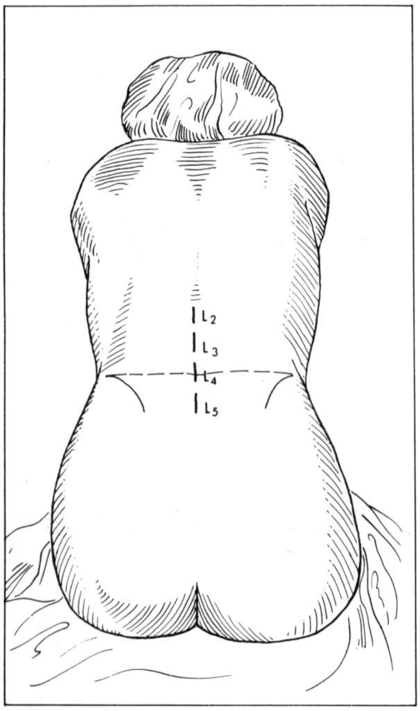

Figure 18. Positioning for Saddle Block

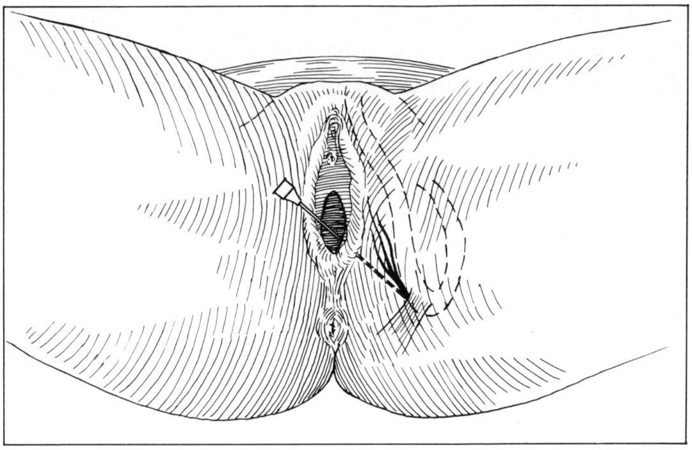

Figure 19. Pudendal Block Infiltration

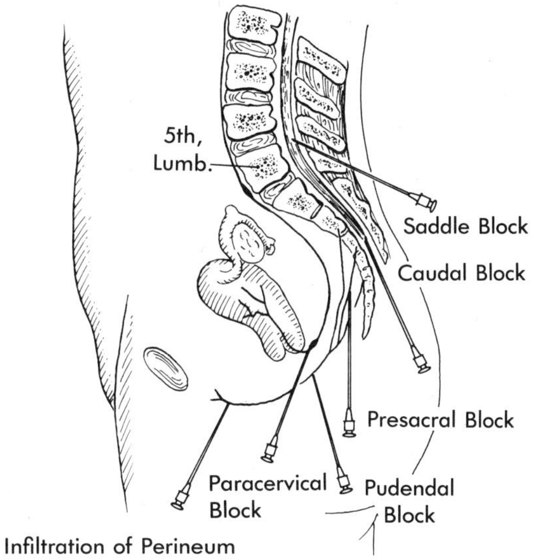

Figure 20. Needle Insertions for Various Regional Anesthesias

24. A patient who receives a continuous caudal anesthesia from the time she is 5 cm. dilated should obtain the following nursing care:

Nursing Care	*Reason for Care*

25. You are asked to set up the delivery room for a patient who is to receive a saddle block anesthesia. List the equipment which you would prepare for the physician to administer the saddle block.

26. Describe your assistance to the patient before, during, and after she receives a saddle block anesthesia.

Before

During

After

27. Check the following statements which apply to pudendal block:

☐ (a) Infiltration of the pudendal nerves with a local anesthetic agent is called a pudendal block.

☐ (b) Xylocaine, 1 per cent is frequently used for a pudendal block.

☐ (c) Uterine contractions are obliterated by a pudendal block.

☐ (d) A pudendal block anesthetizes the perineum and vulva.

☐ (e) A pudendal block is effective for the episiotomy, delivery, and repair of the perineum.

☐ (f) The uterine contractions are not affected by a pudendal block.

☐ (g) A pudendal block relaxes the perineal muscles.

OXYTOCICS

28. Describe the action of oxytocic drugs.

29. Define induction of labor.

30. Name indications for the induction of labor.

31. It is important that the cervix be "ripe" before induction is attempted. What is meant by a "ripe" cervix?

32. Name three oxytocics which may be used for induction.

(a) ______________________________

(b) ______________________________

(c) ______________________________

33. List the nursing responsibilities when caring for a patient who is being induced.

34. Name three oxytocics which are used during the second or third stage of labor to promote uterine contraction following delivery.

(a) ______________________________

(b) ______________________________

(c) ______________________________

35. What is the underlying reason for administering an oxytocic to contract the uterus following delivery?

36. Select the proper classification of the drugs and agents listed in column I from column II.

I			*II*
(a) Cyclopropane	( )	A.	Narcotic analgesic
(b) Demerol	( )	B.	Narcotic antagonist
(c) Ergotrate	( )	C.	Adjunctive tranquilizer
(d) Nitrous oxide	( )	D.	Local anesthetic
(e) Xylocaine	( )	E.	General anesthetic
(f) Lorfan	( )	F.	Oxytocic
(g) Thorazine	( )		
(h) Nisentil	( )		
(i) Pitocin	( )		
(j) Sparine	( )		
(k) Carbocaine	( )		
(l) Nalline	( )		
(m) Syntocinon	( )		
(n) Ether	( )		
(o) Penthrane	( )		
(p) Numorphan	( )		
(q) Trilene	( )		
(r) Methergine	( )		
(s) Phenergan	( )		

Nursing Care During Labor and Delivery

LABOR

Dr. Brewer calls the labor and delivery rooms around 7:30 a.m. to inform you that Mrs. Marilyn Palmer is on her way to the hospital. He tells you that this is her second baby and that her contractions are occurring every seven minutes. He orders an S.S. enema for her on admission.

1. You take Mrs. Palmer's prenatal record from the file and add it to her chart. Which items on the prenatal form should you check in order to be properly informed about Mrs. Palmer?

2. Mr. and Mrs. Palmer arrive at 8:00 a.m. While her husband waits in the fathers' room, you admit Mrs. Palmer. List the items of information pertinent to labor you ask of Mrs. Palmer.

3. What admission procedures do you carry out?

4. If, in your hospital, a perineal prep is given, list the equipment needed, and write down the explanation you give Mrs. Palmer.

Equipment:

Explanation:

5. What is the purpose of giving an S.S. enema to Mrs. Palmer? List the steps you follow in preparing and giving the enema (include explanations and instructions to Mrs. Palmer).

6. An enema is usually contraindicated by the following conditions:

7. Before you gave the enema the resident did a rectal examination. How do you assist in this procedure?

8. After the enema you time Mrs. Palmer's contractions. You find that they are moderate, occur every five minutes, and last 45 seconds. Write down how you:

(a) Ascertain the contractions

(b) Chart your findings on Mrs. Palmer's record

9. Define what is meant by the contractions':

(a) Frequency ______________________________

(b) Duration ______________________________

(c) Intensity ______________________________

10. The fetal heart tones should be listened to between contractions. Why?

11. What is the normal range of fetal heart tones?

12. What deviations in the character of the fetal heart tones would you report to the physician?

13. Outline the nursing care that you will give Mrs. Palmer during the first stage of labor.

You accompany Mr. Palmer to his wife's room. There Dr. Brewer tells him that Mrs. Palmer is 6 cm. dilated and that he expects her to deliver by one o'clock. You notice that Mrs. Palmer seems relieved to see her husband.

14. In what ways do you think Mr. Palmer's presence in the labor room benefits his wife?

15. What can you suggest to him with regard to physical comfort measures? (You have in the meantime given Demerol, 50 mg., and Phenergan, 25 mg. I.M., to Mrs. Palmer.)

16. When Mrs. Palmer reaches 7 cm. dilatation her membranes rupture. How do you comfort Mrs. Palmer physically and emotionally?

17. What specific details will you chart regarding the rupture of the membranes?

18. The period from 7 to 10 cm. dilatation is often referred to as the "transition period." What can you tell Mrs. Palmer about this phase of the first stage?

19. Describe the actual nursing care you and other personnel gave to a recent patient in labor.

20. Describe the patient's reaction to it.

21. List the measures that could have enhanced the patient's experience.

DELIVERY

22. List the basic furniture in the delivery room.

23. Name the essential packs you open in preparation for a delivery.

24. Dr. Brewer asks you to take Mrs. Palmer to the delivery room as soon as she "bulges." Describe "bulging" and its cause.

25. Define "crowning."

26. Describe how you position Mrs. Palmer on the delivery table so Dr. Brewer and his assistant can cleanse and drape the patient.

27. According to Dr. Brewer's instructions you have added to the delivery setup the equipment needed for a pudendal block. List the items you have added.

28. Mrs. Palmer has difficulty panting while Dr. Brewer injects the pudendal block. How can you assist her in carrying out panting?

29. Name and describe the two types of episiotomies most commonly used.

(a) ______________________________

(b) ______________________________

30. Which of the two episiotomies, if extended, may cause a third degree laceration?

31. Which of the two episiotomies is more comfortable for the mother? Why?

IMMEDIATE CARE OF THE NEWBORN

32. Select the item which, immediately following delivery, is most important for the newborn:

☐ (a) To be shown to his parents

☐ (b) To be able to breathe and cry

☐ (c) To have his umbilical cord cut

33. One of the immediate environmental changes for the newborn baby is temperature. Describe how you maintain the warmth of the newborn in your hospital's delivery room.

Appraisal of the newborn should begin the moment the baby is born. Many hospitals now use the Apgar scoring system for making a clinical evaluation of the baby's condition at one minute and five minutes after birth. In the Apgar scoring method five vital signs–heart rate, respiratory effort, muscle tone, reflex irritability, and skin color–are observed and recorded.

Each sign is evaluated according to the degree in which it is present and is given a score of 0, 1, or 2 (see Table 2). The five scores, one given to each of the five signs, are added together for a total score. Apgar scores run from 0 through 10. A score of 10 means a baby is in the best possible condition one minute after birth. Scores of 9, 8, or 7 indicate good condition; 6, 5, or 4 show fair condition; and 3, 2, 1, or 0 indicate poor condition.

Table 2

Sign	*0*	*1*	*2*
I. Heart Rate	Not detectable	Slow (below 100)	Over 100
II. Respiratory effort	Absent	Slow, irregular	Good, crying
III. Muscle tone	Flaccid	Some flexion of extremities	Active motion
IV. Reflex irritability			
1. Response to slap on sole of foot	No response	Grimace	Cry
2. Response to catheter in nostril (tested after oropharynx is clear)	No response	Grimace	Cough or sneeze
V. Color	Blue, pale	Body pink, extremities blue	Completely pink

34. You are assisting with a delivery and have been assigned to record the Apgar score of the newborn. With the help of the Apgar table fill in the score for the newborn who exhibits the following signs:

	Apgar Score
Heart rate over 100	________________
Breathing good, crying	________________
Active motion of legs and arms	________________
Cries in response to slap on sole of foot	________________
Body pink with blue extremities	________________
Total:	________________

35. If the infant's eyes during birth become infected by gonococci, the infection is called ________________ , which may cause ________________ . The prophylactic treatment consists of the administration of ____________ or ________________ .

36. Describe how you administer the treatment named in No. 35.

37. Describe the identification bands used in your hospital. List all the items you are requested to include on the tags before you apply them.

38. Name other means of identification which may be used in addition to identification bands.

39. Before the baby is taken from the delivery room the physician inspects him for abnormalities. What abnormalities may be spotted in the delivery room?

40. In some hospitals one unit of Deladumone (2 cc.) is given to the nonbreast-feeding patient preceding the birth of the baby. What is the action of Deladumone?

41. Why is it best given immediately before delivery?

42. What type of drug is Deladumone?

43. Plan Mrs. Palmer's immediate care following the birth of her baby and the first two hours thereafter. (Don't forget about Mr. Palmer!)

Complications of Labor

1. Name as many reasons as you can think of why a baby may not breathe adequately at the time of birth.

2. List some indications that require extended special attention for the infant (such as placement in the observation nursery or the premature nursery).

3. What is another sign of fetal distress in a cephalic presentation besides a decrease in fetal heart tones?

PREMATURE LABOR

Mrs. Evelyn Green, gr. iii, p. ii, is admitted to the labor rooms with a diagnosis of premature labor. She is in her thirty-fifth week of pregnancy, in active labor, and with her cervix dilated 5 cm.

4. Specify in what ways the management of Mrs. Green's labor will differ from that of a patient at term.

5. How would you adopt the nursing care of Mrs. Green to the factors you stated in No. 4?

6. Mrs. Green asks you: "What are my baby's chances? I am so worried that the baby may be too weak to live." How do you answer Mrs. Green?

UTERINE INERTIA

Mrs. Ruth Jacobs was admitted eight hours ago with regular contractions. During the last three hours no progress of labor has been noted, cervical dilatation still being 4 cm. The physician makes a notation of "secondary uterine inertia" on Mrs. Jacobs' chart and orders: morphine, 10 mg, I.M.; x-ray pelvimetry; and 1000 cc. 5% glucose in water, I.V.

7. Define uterine inertia.

8. Explain the purpose of each of Mrs. Jacobs' orders.

(a) ______________________________

(b) ______________________________

(c) ______________________________

PROLAPSE OF THE CORD

9. What is the danger to the fetus when the umbilical cord prolapses?

10. When is a prolapse of the cord most likely to occur?

11. Describe the essential treatment for prolapse of the cord.

CESAREAN SECTION (see also pages 62–63)

12. Define cesarean section.

13. List the indications for cesarean section.

14. Discuss the statement: Once a cesarean section, always a cesarean section.

15. What is the reason a physician often advises a patient not to have more than three or four pregnancies when cesarean section is the only method by which she can safely deliver?

16. Check the statements which apply to cesarean section:

☐ (a) Patients having elective cesarean section are usually scheduled two weeks prior to their due date in order to prevent the starting of spontaneous labor.

☐ (b) Preparation for cesarean section is the same as for abdominal surgery.

☐ (c) The preoperative medication for cesarean section patients is usually Demerol and Scopolamine.

☐ (d) A catheter inserted before surgery is left open during the operation to drain the bladder and thus prevent trauma to it.

☐ (e) Breast-feeding is contraindicated in a patient having delivered by cesarean section.

☐ (f) Uterine involution in the cesarean section patient is determined by watching the lochial flow, because the patient's abdominal incision would make abdominal palpation painful.

☐ (g) The mother who has had a cesarean section receives postoperative as well as postpartal care.

EMERGENCY DELIVERY

Even in the best-regulated maternity department, it occasionally happens that the patient delivers in the labor room with only the bedside nurse in attendance. When the patient is not delivering under proper aseptic techniques in the delivery room, you should be able to effect safe procedures for the mother's and baby's sakes.

17. The following are some rules which should be observed when an emergency delivery takes place. Give the reason for each principle listed.

Principle	*Reason*
(a) The baby's head should never be forcibly held back.	
(b) If you are the only person present, do not leave the patient to obtain equipment.	
(c) Turn on the call light.	
(d) Help the baby's head deliver slowly by supporting it, and instruct the mother to pant between contractions during delivery of head.	
(e) Keep contaminated articles, including fingers, from the birth canal, and provide as clean a delivery area as possible. Put on sterile gloves if available.	
(f) Hold up the newborn by the feet—no tension on the cord.	
(g) Gently rub the infant's back, if necessary after placing the newborn on the mother's abdomen.	
(h) Wrap the baby in a clean blanket or towels.	
(i) Wait for sterile supplies before cutting the umbilical cord.	
(j) Wait for delivery of placenta until professional help arrives.	

Principle	*Reason*
(k) However, if separation of placenta has occurred, the mother may be asked to bear down to deliver the placenta. The cord and placenta should be supported as they are eased out of the birth canal.	
(l) Save the placenta for later evaluation.	
(m) When the uterus is empty, the fundus should be massaged gently until it is hard.	
(n) Oxytocics may be given with the placenta out of the uterus; if not available, repeat stimulation of the uterus by gently massaging.	

Nursing Care and Teaching during the Puerperium

1. What is understood by the term "postpartum period"?

2. List the changes that occur in the mother's body during this period.

3. Discuss why it is important for a mother to be given the proper care and rest during puerperium.

PHYSICAL CARE

4. List the initial six hours of nursing care for a mother who has just been admitted to the postpartum floor from the recovery room.

After the newly delivered mother has had a chance to rest, she will welcome a bath and perineal care.

5. List the equipment you will bring to the mother's bedside prior to the bath.

6. What explanations will you offer to the mother while giving the bath?

7. In what ways does the postpartum bath and shower differ from the normal?

8. If a patient's perineal stitches are on the left side, you ask her to

turn on her ____________ side while you wash her perineal area. Why?

9. State the purpose for care of perineal sutures.

10. What is accomplished by it?

11. What measures can you employ to relieve the patient's discomfort from perineal sutures?

12. In response to a patient's question on how long her perineal stitches will bother her, you reply (tell the patient the underlying reason for your answer):

13. How soon following delivery is it desirable to have the mother void?

14. In what ways can you encourage spontaneous voiding?

15. What may be the causes for a mother's inability to void?

16. What are the advantages of permitting the patient to be ambulatory within 24 hours after delivery?

17. Explain why primiparas usually do not experience after-pains but many multiparas do.

18. After-pains normally disappear ______ days following delivery.

19. List all the measures which may be indicated for the care of the breasts of the:

Breast-feeding Mother	*Non-breast-feeding Mother*

20. State and describe the cause of engorgement.

21. How soon following delivery may engorgement occur, and how long does it usually last?

One of your responsibilities in caring for the postpartum patient will be the daily inspecting of the patient's nipples, breasts, fundus, lochia, and episiotomy.

22. List the characteristics you look for in each:

(a) Nipples ______________________________

(b) Breasts ______________________________

(c) Fundus ______________________________

(d) Lochia ______________________________

(e) Episiotomy ______________________________

EMOTIONAL ADJUSTMENT

23. Discuss as many factors as possible which can affect the emotional adjustment of the postpartum patient to motherhood.

Factors	*Effect On Mother*

24. How can a new father be made to feel a close member of the family?

FEEDING THE INFANT

Your instructor has discussed with your class the art and practice of breast-feeding. She has stressed that mothers who want to breast-feed need support, encouragement, and personalized practical help. It appears, from a review of many cases, that in most instances, the success or failure of breast-feeding rests on the attitude of the mother as well as the support of her physician and nurses, rather than on the physical make-up of the mother. It is of extreme importance that this fact be recognized by nurses so that success in breast-feeding may be obtained.

25. Now that you are assigned to the postpartum floor, you may expect to care for mothers who choose to breast-feed. In anticipation you prepare an outline for a discussion of breast-feeding with mothers. Write down your topical outline. For example:

(a) Position of mother and baby
(b) Rooting reflex, etc.

On Tuesday morning you are assigned to the rooming-in unit. One of your patients is Mrs. Ruth Toole, a primipara. Her baby, a boy weighing 7 lbs. 6 oz., was born Monday afternoon. From the Kardex you find out that Mrs. Toole is going to breast-feed. As you begin to assist her with morning care, Mrs. Toole asks you if she can hold the baby while you make her bed. After you hand her the baby you encourage her to inspect her child closely. Later on you tell Mrs. Toole that you will be back in time for the baby's first feeding.

26. When you return to Mrs. Toole's room you find out that she would prefer to nurse lying down. You help her to feed from her left breast. Describe how you help Mrs. Toole to a comfortable position.

27. The baby grasps the nipple readily. What is your reason for telling Mrs. Toole to always get the brown pigmented area around the nipple (areola) well into the baby's mouth?

28. While the baby sucks you tell Mrs. Toole the approximate length of time she should nurse today and in the future. (Instruct Mrs. Toole to nurse from one breast or both breasts at each feeding according to your hospital's routine or the pediatrician's order.)

29. At the end of the feeding you show Mrs. Toole the following two ways she may use to get the baby gently off her breast:

(a)

or

(b)

30. You teach Mrs. Toole to "bubble" the baby sitting up. Record verbatim what you say to Mrs. Toole while you assist her.

31. While you are assisting Mrs. Toole her roommate calls you over to help her breast-feed her sleeping baby. What measures do you use trying to wake up the baby?

32. What would you have said to the mother if the baby had not awakened?

33. On her third postpartum day Mrs. Toole's breasts become very heavy and full with milk. Explain how you teach her to support her breast with her hand to get the baby sucking.

34. After the baby started to suck, you notice that the full breast obstructs his breathing. How do you correct this situation?

35. It becomes more comfortable for Mrs. Toole to feed the baby while sitting in a chair. Describe the means you use to position her and the baby correctly.

36. She now bubbles the baby halfway through the feeding and at the end. You already taught Mrs. Toole one way of bubbling. Now you teach her a second method whereby she holds the baby over her shoulder. State your instructions.

37. What can you tell Mrs. Toole about the relationship between emptying the breasts by feeding the baby and the amount of milk produced?

38. Mrs. Toole is quite concerned about "drippings" from her breasts between feedings. Can you offer her some help?

39. To prevent sore nipples you advise Mrs. Toole to "air" her breasts. What does this mean?

40. If Mrs. Toole has developed sore nipples, what measures would have been useful to her?

41. Mrs. Betty Cross is another patient assigned to you in the rooming-in unit. She is bottle-feeding her baby. Describe how you teach her to test the temperature of the formula and the flow of milk from the nipple.

42. List the pointers you give Mrs. Cross regarding the placing and holding of the bottle.

43. Mrs. Cross plans to use a commercial formula service (home delivery) when she leaves the hospital. Her baby is on liquid Enfamil (1:1 strength) formula. She worries about what might happen if she runs out of formula at home. She also wants your advice about getting a supply of formula when spending the weekends at their country cottage. Mrs. Cross says she does not want to be bothered making formula. What are you advising?

44. Before lunchtime you sit down in your patients' room to chat with them. The talk gets around to the topic of how often to feed the baby and how one knows when the baby has had enough. You answer the questions and decide to add a word about the atmosphere conducive to happy feeding times and the benefits accruing from it to the baby and mother. Record your answers and advice.

45. Study the following nursing care plan. Enter under *Nursing Observations* the steps you would take to verify the listed *Needs and Problems.* Indicate under *Nursing Interventions* the care you would give Mrs. Gillian to relieve her needs and problems.

NURSING CARE PLAN

Name: Mrs. Edith Gillian Rm. 418

3rd day postpartum

Age: 29

Gr. iii, p. iii

Boy: 7 lbs. 9 oz.

Low forceps

Episiotomy

Bottle feeding

Medical Orders:

Up ad lib

General diet

Sitz bath prn

Nupercainal ointment

MOM 30 cc. hs prn

SS enema prn

Codeine 30 mg.
Aspirin 0.60 gm. q 4 hrs prn

Tace 12 mg. bid for 5 days

Seconal 100 mg. hs prn

Needs and Problems:	*Nursing Observations:*
(a) Complains of after-pains and painful suture area.	(a)
(b) Engorgement of breasts.	(b)
(c) Has not yet moved bowels.	(c)
(d) "Postpartum blues"	(d)

Nursing Intervention:

(a)

(b)

(c)

(d)

GUIDANCE IN CARE OF NEWBORN

46. The census of the postpartum unit is 27 delivered mothers, 12 primiparas and 15 multiparas. Group instruction on bathing the baby and formula preparation is given twice weekly. You and your classmates would like to offer some additional discussions, and you, therefore, ask the mothers to suggest topics of interest to them. List the topics you anticipate the group to propose, or that you may want to suggest:

47. In preparation for teaching the baby bath and formula-making classes, outline two discussions with all the specific, salient points you need to teach. Include the listing of equipment.

Baby Bath

(Use doll or baby)

Equipment:

Outline of discussion:

Formula Preparation

(Terminal method)

Equipment:

Outline of discussion:

48. What are some of the emotions which mothers experience who have had a stillbirth or whose babies have died shortly following birth?

49. In which ways can you be helpful to a grieving mother?

Complications of the Puerperium

1. Name the three leading causes of maternal mortality.

(a) ______________________________

(b) ______________________________

(c) ______________________________

2. For each mortality cause listed, state prophylactic and/or therapeutic measures used against it.

(a) ______________________________

(b) ______________________________

(c) ______________________________

3. Complete the following listings of postpartum complications (be thorough).

POSTPARTUM HEMORRHAGE

Contributing Causes	*Symptoms*	*Treatment*

PUERPERAL INFECTION

Contributing Causes	*Symptoms*	*Treatment*

MASTITIS

Contributing Causes	*Symptoms*	*Treatment*

THROMBOPHLEBITIS

Contributing Causes	*Symptoms*	*Treatment*

Characteristics and Nursing Care of the Newborn Baby

INFANT MORTALITY

For all its wealth and scientific progress, the United States ranks below at least eleven other nations in its ability to help infants survive their first year of life. During those first twelve months, 23.8 out of every 1000 American babies die, compared with 12.6 in Sweden, 14.7 in the Netherlands, and so forth.

1. Cite factors which account for the relatively high American infant mortality.

2. How could the nation's infant mortality rate be reduced?

3. Discuss the statement: There is a limit beyond which infant mortality cannot be reduced.

4. Draw a blueprint for a nursery that is to accommodate 12 cribs. State the distance between cribs. Specify where door(s), sinks, and the like, are located. Describe how each operates. Include all equipment, such as receptacles for dirty diapers, oxygen outlets, and so forth. (If you like, number each item and then identify each number in a legend.)

HANDWASHING

5. Briefly discuss the purpose of the handwashing technique in the nursery.

6. List the steps of the handwashing procedure used in your hospital.

7. Discuss the instances when you must wash your hands in the nursery.

INITIAL CARE

8. Miss Cline, delivery room nurse, enters the nursery with a newborn baby for admission. List the items to be checked together with Miss Cline in receiving the baby.

9. While placing the baby in his crib, you carefully check the conditions of the following:

(a) ______________________________

(b) ______________________________

(c) ______________________________

10. Describe the steps you follow when weighing the newborn.

11. Many hospitals lower the head of the baby's crib for the first 24 hours following birth. What is the purpose of this positioning?

12. A sterile rubber bulb syringe is placed in the crib to be available for removing excess mucus from the baby's throat and mouth. Describe explicitly how you handle the bulb syringe when removing mucus from the baby's mouth.

While you give baby Smith his initial bath, Mr. Smith watches through the nursery window. He starts talking to you, and, using the intercom system (foot operated), you have the following conversation with him. (Remember to include in your replies the reasons underlying your answers.)

13. Mr. Smith: "Is it normal for the baby to keep his arms and legs drawn up?"

Your reply:

14. Mr. Smith: "His fingers seem kind of bluish. Is he cold?"

Your reply:

15. Mr. Smith: "The baby's head is pointed rather than round. Is something wrong with him?"

Your reply:

16. Mr. Smith: "When you bumped against the crib the baby got so scared. Is it all right for him to throw his arms out like that?"

Your reply:

17. Mr. Smith: "Why is that pin attached to his belly?"
Your reply:

18. Mr. Smith, laughing when the baby voids: "He got you all wet; what a boy! My wife and I want the baby circumcised. When will that be done?"
Your reply:

19. Mr. Smith: "My wife is going to bottle-feed. When will the baby get his first bottle? And then, how often will he be fed?"
Your reply:

20. Mr. Smith: "Do you always wrap the babies up like that in a blanket?"
Your reply:

The following descriptions (No. 21 to 25) are normal reflexes of the newborn. Identify them:

21. Gentle stimulation of the sole of the baby's foot causes extension and moderate abduction of the big toe, whereas the other toes flex:

____

22. When the baby's head is turned to one side, the extremities on the same side extend; those on the opposite side flex:

____

23. When the infant is startled by jarring of the crib or a loud noise, he draws his legs up and brings his arms around his chest as if in an embrace:

____

24. When a finger or other object is placed into his hand, the infant grasps and holds it:

____

25. The baby will make crawling movements when placed on his abdomen and stepping movements when supported in an upright position:

____

26. State how you will instruct Mrs. Smith in the home care of the umbilical cord.

27. State the nursery nurse's responsibilities preceding a circumcision.

28. Describe the nursing care following the circumcision.

29. What will you tell Mrs. Smith concerning the home care of her baby's circumcision?

CHARACTERISTICS AND ACTIVITIES

There are certain characteristics and activities of the newborn which must be closely observed by the nurse to insure the infant's well-being. Sketched in the diagram are the conditions of which the nurse must be particularly cognizant.

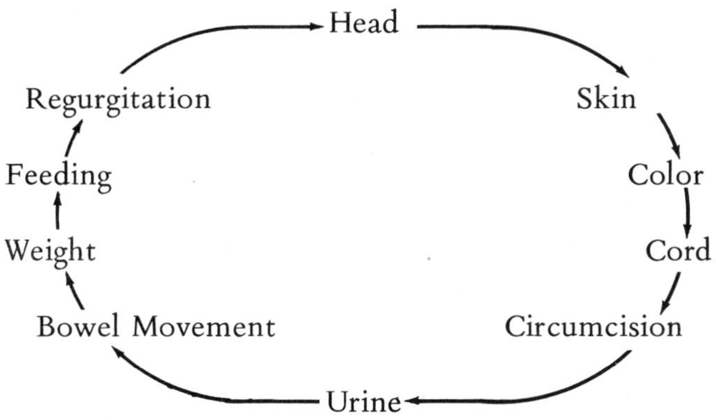

Head

In the foregoing conversation Mr. Smith commented on the elongated head of his baby following birth.

30. The head's accommodation to the birth canal is called ____________ ____________. When does it disappear? ____________

31. Edema of the scalp, a soft swelling on the head resulting from pressure on the scalp veins where the head of the fetus met the resistance of the cervix during the birth process, is called ____________. It generally disappears within ____________ after birth.

32. A soft spongy mass over one of the skull bones caused by bleeding under the periosteum is called ____________. It is due to trauma during delivery. How long does it persist? ____________

33. The infant at birth has well defined fontanels. Complete the following:

	Shape	*Closure*
(a) Anterior fontanel	____________	____________
(b) Posterior fontanel	____________	____________

34. A sunken anterior fontanel in an infant indicates ____________.

35. A bulging anterior fontanel is a sign of ____________ ____________.

Skin

36. Check which of the following descriptions apply to the newborn's skin:

☐ (a) Peeling of the baby's epidermis during the first week is normal.

☐ (b) Dryness is a characteristic of the newborn's skin, with fissures at the wrist and ankles not uncommon.

☐ (c) Plugged-up sebaceous glands, called milia, may be seen over the nose and chin during the first two weeks.

Color

In addition to cyanosis, the baby's color is carefully observed for evidence of jaundice.

37. The most common form of jaundice in the newborn is caused by the rapid destruction of extra red blood cells. This type of jaundice is called ____________. When does it become evident?

38. What is the treatment for this type of jaundice?

39. If a mother asks you about the duration of this jaundice, what will you tell her?

40. Jaundice that occurs during the first 48 hours and has no normal cause is called ______________________.

41. State its most common cause.

____

42. Discuss why this type of jaundice should be reported to the physician at once.

Weight

43. When does physiologic weight loss occur in the infant?

44. How much weight loss is within normal limits?

45. What factors contribute to the weight loss?

46. Discuss when the infant's weight normally becomes stationary and his birth weight is regained.

47. State how you would describe to a mother the normal weight gain over the first year.

Urine

48. The newborn is expected to void within ______________ following birth.

49. What is your reply to a mother who asks you how often her baby will wet his diapers when she returns home?

50. How many diapers per day would you recommend a mother to order when using diaper service?

51. Would you advise this mother to also buy some diapers? If so, how many?

52. A mother who does not use a diaper service should have about ____ diapers on hand.

Bowel Movement

53. Define meconium.

54. State the characteristics of the stools of breast-fed babies and formula-fed babies.

Stool	*Color*	*Consistency*	*Frequency*
(a) Breast-fed baby			
(b) Formula-fed baby			

Feeding

Human and cow's milk are basically not too dissimilar; both depend to some extent on intake. Most formulas that are made from modified cow's milk are adjusted to the composition of breast milk by an increase in carbohydrate content.

55. To supply 20 calories per ounce, liquid formulas are diluted with

______ parts of water. This results in a ______________ strength.

56. To supply 20 calories per ounce, ________________ of powdered

formula is diluted in ________________________ of water. This results

in a ______________ strength.

57. Dr. Hem orders 24 oz. of liquid Similac formula (1:1 strength) per day for baby Smith. In preparing the formula how much Similac will you use and how much water?

58. For baby Powel Dr. Hem orders 24 oz. of powdered Similac formula (1:2 strength) per day. In preparing the formula how much powdered Similac will you use and how much water?

The average daily caloric requirement for the full-term infant is approximately 50 to 55 calories per pound of body weight. The fluid requirement ranges from 2 to 3 ounces per pound of body weight in a 24-hour period.

59. Baby Crown weighs 6½ lbs. Figuring 55 calories per pound of body weight and 3 ounces of fluid requirement per pound of body weight, what are the 24-hour caloric and fluid requirements of baby Crown? (Show your calculations.)

(a) 24-hour caloric requirement:

(b) 24-hour fluid requirement:

Regurgitation

60. Define regurgitation.

61. What is it caused by?

62. List the measures that may reduce regurgitation.

TESTING FOR PHENYLKETONURIA (PKU)

63. Which method (test) is used in your hospital to test the newborn for PKU? ________________________ On which principle is this test based?

64. How would you define PKU to a mother and the reason for testing infants for it?

ABNORMALITIES AND DISEASES OF THE NEWBORN INFANT

1. Abnormalities and diseases of the newborn may be classified into the following categories. Give as many examples of each as you can.

Categories *Examples*

Congenital malformations:

Birth injuries:

Respiratory diseases:

Infections:

Miscellaneous disturbances:

CONGENITAL HEART DISEASE

2. List the symptoms accompanying congenital heart disease.

3. What nursing measures can you anticipate when the diagnosis of congenital heart disease is made?

4. What treatment is available for babies with congenital heart disease?

HYDROCEPHALUS

Baby Wenger was born three days ago, the first child of Mr. and Mrs. Ernest Wenger. At birth both the obstetrician and pediatrician were suspicious of the size of the baby's head. Daily measurements of the head's circumference revealed increases of 0.3 cm. on each of the three days following birth. A tentative diagnosis of hydrocephalus was then made.

5. Define hydrocephalus.

6. What types of treatment may be used for it?

7. What is the prognosis for children with hydrocephalus?

8. State the measures and precautions which you teach Mrs. Wenger before discharge to help her take care of her baby at home.

ANENCEPHALY

9. Define anencephaly.

10. Why is this condition incompatible with life?

DOWN'S SYNDROME

When baby Klein was born, the delivery-room nurse became suspicious of the baby's appearance. She noticed the baby's flat head and face, and slanted eyes. On careful examination the obstetrician made the diagnosis of probable mongolism (a definite diagnosis was to be made following chromosome studies).

11. What signs characteristic of mongolism could the obstetrician have possibly found in addition to the ones observed by the nurse?

12. State the three types of Down's syndrome which may be revealed by chromosome studies:

(a) ______________________________

(b) ______________________________

(c) ______________________________

13. Discuss the relationship of chromosome studies and genetic counseling, and how these measures can help parents in their decision on future childbearing.

Baby Klein's disorder was diagnosed as Down's syndrome due to an abnormal number of chromosomes, 47 instead of 46. The Kleins have two other children, a boy 12 years old and a girl 7 years of age. Mrs. Klein is 44 years old, Mr. Klein 50.

The Kleins' obstetrician discussed with them the probable potentials of their newborn baby. The obstetrician indicated that he favored early institutionalization for the baby. The Kleins were undecided.

14. What factors do you suppose will influence the Kleins' decision on institutionalization versus home care?

15. What institutional facilities are available in your community? Are these private or public facilities?

16. Following your inquiries concerning the availability of institutional facilities, discuss cost and quality of care.

17. Discuss your own feelings concerning home care and institutional care for a baby with Down's syndrome. What influences your attitude?

There are many ambivalent emotions parents experience when faced with a baby exhibiting characteristics which interfere with a normal growth pattern.

18. Discuss what some of these emotions may be.

19. In what ways can you, as a nurse, help parents such as the Kleins express their dilemma?

20. State various approaches you could use to start the conversation in case Mrs. Klein does not bring up the subject (and you feel it is not contraindicated to talk with her about it).

21. Basing your answers on the actual home situation of the Kleins and their community resources, what kind of affirmative response could you give Mrs. Klein concerning:

(a) Home care of the child

(b) Institutionalizing of the child

22. Describe the care of the baby for the first few months that should be familiar to Mrs. Klein in case the baby goes home with her.

CLEFT LIP AND PALATE

23. Define cleft lip.

24. Define cleft palate.

25. Before feeding a baby with cleft lip and palate you have to select a suitable nipple. What types of nipples are available and what do they accomplish?

26. List the instructions you would give a mother who has a baby with cleft lip and palate. This information is for the interim of eight weeks following discharge, after which she will bring the baby back for surgical repair of the harelip.

27. Describe supportive measures you could discuss with this mother to deal with her environmental and family situations (this is her first baby).

28. At what age is a cleft palate usually repaired?

CLUBFOOT

29. Write down the areas of care you feel need discussion with a mother who is taking home her five-day-old baby who has a clubfoot. The baby wears a cast on his left foot and leg up to his knee. The cast will not be changed until the baby is four weeks old.

INTRACRANIAL HEMORRHAGE

30. List some causes of intracranial hemorrhage.

31. List the symptoms of intracranial hemorrhage.

32. Describe the care of a newborn diagnosed as having intracranial hemorrhage.

33. What factors influence the prognosis of a baby having intracranial hemorrhage?

RESPIRATORY DISTRESS DISEASE

34. Discuss what is known at present about the cause of respiratory distress disease.

35. Careful observation of all newborns is the responsibility of the nurse. Which babies in particular would you watch for symptoms of respiratory distress disease? Why?

36. What are some of the symptoms exhibited by babies having respiratory distress disease?

37. What is the treatment for respiratory distress disease?

PNEUMONIA

38. List contributory causes to pneumonia in the newborn.

39. Name some preventive measures to avoid pneumonia in the newborn.

40. Describe the treatment for pneumonia.

INFECTIONS

41. Discuss the ways infections may be acquired in utero, during birth, and following delivery. Include a discussion of the implications which infections can have on the fetus and newborn.

42. What preventive and prophylactic measures may reduce the incidence of infections?

THRUSH

43. Name the causes of thrush.

44. List its symptoms.

45. Describe fully the care and prognosis of a newborn having contracted thrush.

46. How would you explain thrush to a mother whose baby has the infection, and how would you describe to her the treatment given in the hospital?

47. What sanitary measures would you teach the mother?

DIARRHEA

48. What are the symptoms of diarrhea?

49. Name some causative organisms.

50. Give the reasons in column II for the treatment of diarrhea listed in column I:

I	*II*
(a) Stool culture	______________________
(b) Parenteral fluids or clysis	______________________
(c) Weak tea or Casec water	______________________
(d) Antibiotics	______________________
(e) Strict isolation	______________________

51. Is a diarrheal outbreak in a newborn nursery considered a serious complication? Why?

52. Describe the measures used to prevent an epidemic of diarrhea in a newborn nursery where three cases of diarrhea have been diagnosed.

ERYTHROBLASTOSIS FETALIS

53. Explain what is accomplished by an exchange transfusion of the newborn in:

(a) Rh incompatibility

(b) ABO incompatibility

54. In general terms discuss the reliance on laboratory findings (Coombs test, bilirubin, and hemoglobin determination) when making a decision to perform an exchange transfusion.

55. What are the physical characteristics exhibited by a newborn for whom an exchange transfusion is indicated?

56. Define kernicterus. Why is it an irreversible condition?

57. Explain why ABO incompatibility may afflict the first-born baby, whereas Rh incompatibility is usually first exhibited by the second or third baby.

58. Describe how you care for the umbilical cords of babies born to Rh-negative mothers in your hospital.

59. You have been asked to help with an exchange transfusion. The blood for the transfusion, a normal saline solution, I. V. tubing, the instrument trays and drugs used during the procedure, and an oxygen mask and flowmeter are set up. You are asked to listen to the baby's heartbeat and to fasten the stethoscope to the baby's chest for the duration of the exchange transfusion. Describe exactly how you proceed to do this.

60. Next you are asked to position the baby for the exchange transfusion. Describe the method used in your hospital to restrain the baby.

61. You have the responsibility of keeping a record of the amount of blood infused and withdrawn. The physician, after threading the catheter into the umbilical vein, proceeds to exchange in units of 10 cc. What does this mean?

62. On the tally sheet (page 157) indicate how you record a withdrawal of 290 cc. of blood and an infusion of 280 cc. of blood. Underline in red the intervals at which you notify the physician of the amounts withdrawn and infused.

63. What is the reason for notifying the physician at the underlined intervals?

64. Write down on the tally sheet (page 157) the action (if any) taken at these intervals.

65. What is the reason for rinsing the syringes used during an exchange transfusion in normal saline to which heparin has been added?

66. Outline the nursing care of the newborn for the first 24 hours following an exchange transfusion.

After you assist with the exchange transfusion and the baby has been returned to the nursery (baby withstood the procedure well), you visit the mother of the infant in her room. She is tense and tells you that the physician has told her that the exchange transfusion went well.

67. List questions and topics of conversation relating to the baby and the transfusion procedure which you could bring up in order to make sure that the mother has an accurate knowledge of what has happened, and also the satisfaction of knowing that the best was done for her infant.

68. The following day you find out that the baby does not need a repeat exchange transfusion. What can you tell the mother about the prognosis and future development of her baby?

EXCHANGE TRANSFUSION SHEET

In	*Out*	*Total*	*Comments*

Phototherapy and the Newborn

The practice of treating hyperbilirubinemia in newborn infants by phototherapy has increased in recent years. According to the 1972 annual report of the National Research Council's Division of Medical Sciences, phototherapy has largely replaced other methods of treatment because of its simplicity of application: the infants, their eyes shielded, are placed under lights for varying periods during the first week after birth. The report estimates that from 10,000 to 35,000 babies may be exposed to this treatment annually.

However, the report states that the scientific and technical bases of this practice are inadequate. There are insufficient data on the biologic effects of phototherapy on newborn infants; a suitable dose response curve has not been constructed; the most beneficial (and least harmful) type of light has not been defined or developed; and the mechanical equipment for applying the light and measuring the effective therapeutic dose delivered is inadequate.

Accordingly, the Division of Medical Sciences is conducting a two-year investigation of the subject under the direction of a multidisciplinary Committee on Phototherapy in the Newborn, comprised of pediatricians, photobiologists, and bioengineers. It aims to develop guidelines for correct medical practice, stimulate research, and encourage the development of safe and efficacious equipment. Sponsored by a grant from the United States Maternal and Child Health Service, the Committee plans to complete its work in 1974.

By now the effectiveness of phototherapy in the treatment of hyperbilirubinemia seems well established. According to the latest studies, continuous phototherapy during the first four days of life seems significantly superior to intermittent phototherapy in lowering the concentration of serum bilirubin. However, while its use is recommended for infants with serum bilirubin concentrations of 10 mg. per 100 ml. or higher, in the case of an infant whose clinical condition predisposes him to kernicterus, phototherapy should be used earlier but not in place of exchange transfusion.

Bilirubin levels should be monitored for two or three days after phototherapy in order to detect failure or rebound.

69. State the areas in which guidelines for the use of phototherapy in hyperbilirubinemia are indicated.

70. If phototherapy proves to be an effective and safe means of treating hyperbilirubinemia, list its advantages.

71. State the conditions which would necessitate an exchange transfusion in spite of the newborn's treatment with phototherapy.

THE NEWBORN OF A DIABETIC MOTHER

72. Describe the appearance and characteristics that a baby born to a diabetic mother may exhibit.

73. To what postnatal complication is the baby born to a diabetic mother especially prone?

74. Explain why babies of diabetic mothers are often delivered by either induction or cesarean section.

75. Discuss why the fetal and neonatal mortality rates of babies born to diabetic mothers are higher than those of other babies.

You notice that the actual weight loss of a baby born to a diabetic mother is greater than the physiologic weight loss (10% of body weight) on his third day.

76. What action do you take? Why?

77. What measures are taken at the time of delivery and thereafter to prevent respiratory distress?

78. Describe in what ways the care of a newborn of a diabetic mother differs from the care usually given.

79. What is the baby's prognosis if he progresses without complications during the first week?

SICKLE CELL DISEASE

Many Americans heard of sickle cell disease for the first time in 1971, when the government allocated funds for research and treatment of this severe and incapacitating blood disorder that affects about one in every 500 black babies born in the United States each year. Even within the black communities of this country there has been little dissemination of information about this condition and its hereditary aspects.

Sickle cell anemia is an inherited disease that affects black people almost exclusively. Accompanied by severe anemia and by recurrent painful episodes called "crises," the disease markedly reduces life expectancy. It is unusual for a person with the disease to live beyond the third decade, and indeed many die during infancy and childhood. Estimates indicate that as many as 45,000 to 75,000 black people in the United States may have sickle cell anemia; thus the incidence of the disease is six times greater than that of cystic fibrosis and 20 times higher than that of phenylketonuria (PKU). More than two million are said to be carriers of the genetic sickle hemoglobin trait.

Techniques are available to diagnose the disease and differentiate between those who have sickle cell anemia and those who carry the trait. Large-scale testing of school children and adults is now being initiated so that those who have the disease or are carriers can be taught how to try to prevent crises and avoid stressful situations. It has been found that a crisis may be triggered by preceding viral or bacterial infections, a cold, hypoxia, or stress situations (trauma, strenuous physical exertion, emotional stress, and extreme fatigue). Genetic counseling is widely endorsed since when people choose to marry to have children they have a right to know what the facts are.

Each person inherits two sets of genes, one from each parent. A person with sickle cell anemia has inherited a sickle cell gene from each parent. A person who inherits a sickle cell gene from only one parent is called a trait. Thus it requires two traits to produce a child with sickle cell anemia, and the odds are one in four for such a birth. The chances of producing another trait are one in two. One child in four will inherit all normal hemoglobin and thus be free of the disease. If only one parent carries the sickle cell trait, two children in four risk having it, and two in four can be expected to be normal. The odds of this genetic roulette apply to each birth.

The disease is caused by a defect in the hemoglobin molecules within the red blood cells, which carry oxygen throughout the body. Each hemoglobin molecule contains 574 amino acids. In sickle cell hemoglobin, two of these amino acids are replaced by two others. At the basic level, the change is so small that one might be inclined to ignore it, yet for the individual, it is a matter of life and death.

When sickle cell hemoglobin is deprived of oxygen, the red blood cells lose their round, doughnut-like shape and take on a sickle or quarter-moon appearance. In this condition the red blood cells are unable to pass through the body's capillaries. The cells jam up like leaves clogging a drainpipe. As a result tissue is deprived of the oxygen it needs and dies. This painful event is called a "crisis."

In crisis, a person suddenly develops intense pain—usually in the abdomen, back, chest, hips, arms, or legs. The heart may be partly or fatally damaged, or a stroke may result. Sickle cell sufferers are extremely vulnerable to infection, particularly to pneumonia, and many develop skin ulcers at the ankle.

Women with the sickle cell trait have a higher incidence of urinary infection during pregnancy, and traits sometimes pass blood in their urine.

The disease results from a gene mutation that occurred centuries ago in Africa, and which became common because it offered a protection against malaria. For some unknown reason, malarial parasites cannot survive in sickled red blood cells. In the United States and other areas where malaria has been eradicated, sickle cell trait is no longer an advantage.

Sickled red cells are fragile and are rapidly destroyed in the circulation. Their life span may be only 30 to 40 days, instead of the normal 120 days. Although the person with sickle cell anemia can produce new cells at a rapid rate, he becomes anemic because the rate of destruction of cells is greater than that of production.

In a person with sickle cell trait, 35 to 40 per cent of hemoglobin in the red blood cells is the abnormal hemoglobin S. Spontaneous sickling does not occur in the circulation because the red cells contain enough normal hemoglobin A to counteract the effects of the hemoglobin S. There is no disease or anemia associated with sickle cell trait, and the trait does not affect life expectancy or fertility. In fact, an affected person probably never knows that he has the sickle cell trait and is a carrier of the sickle gene unless special blood tests are conducted. The problem arises when two traits produce a child who inherits the disease.

At the present time treatment of the disease is largely experimental. The chemical urea has been used to reverse sickling once crisis has begun, but this compound is far from innocuous. Massive diuresis (20 to 30 liters of urine) may occur over a treatment period of 24 to 36 hours, as well as multiple other serious side effects. Some investigators are experimenting with potassium cyanate, an inhibitor of sickling.

The ultimate cure may be found along unexpected paths (as it was with RhoGAM, the "vaccine" for Rh-negative mothers). The intensive research now being conducted raises the hope that a preventive factor may be found for this debilitating disease.

80. Mr. James Douglas carries the sickle cell trait, but his wife Dorothy is not a trait. Upon their request their physician furnishes them with the possibilities of inheritance. Show on Figure 21A the possible outcome of a pregnancy.

81. Mr. and Mrs. James Alexander are both sickle cell traits. Upon genetic counseling they are advised of the possible outcome of a pregnancy. Indicate on Figure 21B what they were told.

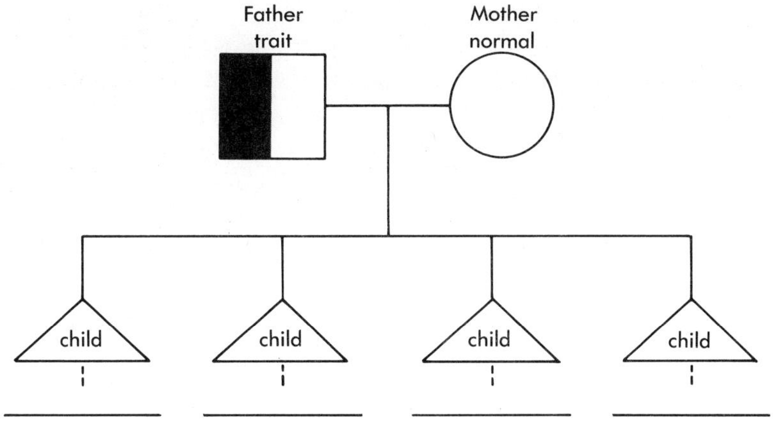

A. On the lines provided, indicate the possible inheritance.

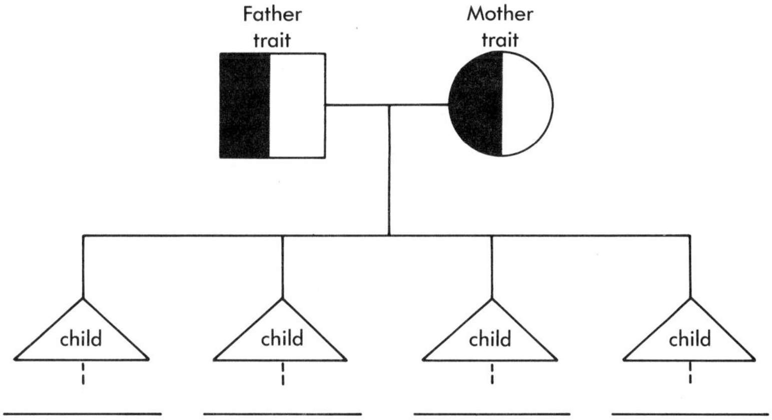

B. On the lines provided, indicate the possible inheritance.

Figure 21. Sickle Cell Inheritance

Characteristics and Nursing Care

1. What is the American Academy of Pediatrics' definition of a premature baby?

2. What is meant by a low-birth-weight infant?

3. List factors which may contribute toward prematurity.

4. Name the characteristics and symptoms of a premature baby.

Mrs. Janet Bradly gives birth to her first child during her thirty-fourth week of pregnancy. The boy weighs 3 lbs. 4 oz. at birth and is placed in an incubator. The pediatrician tells Mr. and Mrs. Bradly that the boy's condition needs careful observation during the next few days. He encourages the couple to go to the nursery to see their infant.

5. Describe the benefits which baby Bradly derives from being placed in an incubator.

6. The immediate nursing care for baby Bradly involves:

7. Baby Bradly is not receiving oxygen therapy. However, if he were, you would have to measure the oxygen content within the incubator at regular intervals. List the steps you follow when using the oxygen analyzer in your hospital.

8. Why is it important to know and control the amount of oxygen administered to a premature baby?

9. Mrs. Bradly sleeps for a few hours after she is brought to the post-partum floor from the delivery room suite. When her husband returns to visit her, you offer to take Mrs. Bradly in a wheelchair to the nursery window so the couple can see their infant together. While assisting Mrs. Bradly into the wheelchair, you prepare the parents for the nursery visit by describing their son and his immediate environment. Write down your description.

10. Name some of the thoughts and feelings which you think might cross Mr. and Mrs. Bradly's minds as they see the baby, and during the next few days.

It is generally recognized that if parents are allowed to express their thoughts and are supported by hospital personnel, they are able to cope positively with the demands and responsibilities placed upon them by a premature baby.

11. State what you as a nurse can do for the Bradlys and other parents in similar situations to support the foregoing statement.

When baby Bradly is 36 hours old he is fed 5% Dextrose water with a special premature bottle and nipple. Because he sucks well and retains his feeding, he is started on ½ ounce of Olac formula every two to three hours.

12. Why is a premie fed more often and smaller amounts than a normal newborn?

13. Name means other than the special premature bottle and nipple that can be used to feed the premature baby. What determines the method used?

Baby Bradly's condition remains satisfactory. When Mrs. Bradly is discharged on the sixth postpartum day, the pediatrician tells the Bradlys that he will probably keep the baby in the hospital for another six to eight weeks. He explains to the parents that by then he expects the baby to weigh five pounds and be strong enough to be taken care of at home. He asks the parents to call him or the nursery for progress reports about the baby.

14. On her discharge day Mrs. Bradly comments to you that the thought of six to eight weeks without the baby at home gives her such a letdown feeling. Although you lead Mrs. Bradly to understand that you know how she feels, you also try to point out the positive aspects of this period. Name some of them.

15. Does your hospital provide any direct teaching sessions for mothers before their premature babies are discharged to them? If so, describe them, and explain whether or not you believe that the type of instruction and assistance given meets the mothers' needs.

16. If your hospital has no definite teaching period set up, outline a teaching plan (topics to be taught and discussed, and how) that would be of help to Mrs. Bradly before she takes the baby home. Plan for these instructions to start four weeks postpartum.

GUIDANCE IN FAMILY PLANNING

Birth is remarkable all the more so because the reproductive organs, having performed an enormous task, very soon return to their former size and functions. Within about a month they are ready to begin their work again. The first ovulation after delivery is likely to occur about this time. Although breast-feeding may hasten the return of the reproductive organs to their original size and may delay menstruation, it will not prevent ovulation, as many people believe.

Therefore, conception can occur before the first menstrual period after delivery. Most often the first period occurs about 6 weeks after delivery. At this time the mother will be returning to her physician for her "6 weeks" examination. Unless she wishes another pregnancy to follow very soon, it is essential at this time to discuss with her physician the method of conception control recommended for her. Even if she has used a method at an earlier time, it must now be re-evaluated in view of the physical changes of child-bearing.

Nursing is currently recognizing that family planning is an integral part of comprehensive maternity care. Counseling in contraception is as natural to family care as counseling about immunization, good nutrition, or chest x-rays.

However, many nurses have hesitated to discuss family planning with patients because they felt the decision was a matter for each family to decide. So it is. But freedom to choose requires knowledge of the choices. Only when men and women know what family planning is and where it can be obtained do they protect their right to choose freely. If the nurse withholds this type of information she is in a sense deciding negatively for them.

Ignorance of safe methods for conception control places a heavy burden on the mental and physical health of those mothers who bear more children than they desire or can adequately care for. It is wise to remember that family planning takes into account economic as well as health factors.

Many hospitals and health departments include birth control information in their classes for expectant parents. Knowledge that they can space their children's births can be a great comfort to couples awaiting a child – whether this is the first or the fourth.

The period just before and after delivery is so appropriate for counseling that some hospitals assign a nurse to visit each new mother during her stay to discuss family planning at the bedside. Group lecture-discussions are also offered in some large hospitals and films are shown to groups of patients with a nurse on hand to answer questions.

Many valid approaches can be used on an individual basis. The simplest– "Do you wish help in planning your family?" or "Would you like to obtain birth control information?"–is probably the most effective in most situations. If a less direct opening is desired, the nurse may ask, "How soon would you like to have your next baby?" This will often elicit "not for a long time," or "not for a year or two anyway," or even "never, I hope." This gives the nurse an opportunity to ask, "Do you know what family planning methods are available? Do you need any help? Do you know where to get it?"

METHODS OF CONTRACEPTION

Generally, methods of birth control can be grouped under nonsurgical and surgical methods. In order of effectiveness, nonsurgical methods are grouped as follows:

Oral contraceptives (the pill): 0.0 to 0.2% failure
Intra-uterine devices: 1 to 4% failure
Diaphragm: 2 to 8% failure
Spermicidal jellies, foams, and tablets: 8 to 30% failure
Rhythm: 15 to 30% failure

Surgical methods are:

Hysterectomy
Bilateral tubal ligation
Laparoscopy
Ovariotexy
Vasectomy
Reversible male sterilization

Nonsurgical Contraceptive Methods

Oral Contraceptives. One tablet is taken each day for 20 days, starting on the fifth day of the menstrual cycle. The medication suppresses anterior pituitary secretion of gonadotropins, thereby inhibiting ovulation. It also has a direct stimulating effect on the endometrium, so that from one to four days after the last tablet is taken the endometrium sloughs and bleeds as a result of hormonal withdrawal. The bleeding usually is less profuse than that of a normal period and may last only two or three days. Some women have no bleeding at all. The patient starts taking the medication again on the fifth day of the cycle, or seven days after she has taken the last pill if she does not bleed, and continues for another 20 days. This can be continued indefinitely.

If contraceptive tablets are taken according to the recommended schedule, the incidence of unplanned pregnancy should be close to zero. If they are taken irregularly during the cycle, ovulation and fertilization may occur. With further improvements, such as the one-month or three-month pill, oral contraception will undoubtedly become the most widely used of all methods.

Intra-uterine devices. IUCDs are small objects in the shape of a ring, loop, coil, or bow made of plastic or stainless steel. They are inserted into the uterus by the physician and may be left in place indefinitely. Nylon tabs hang outside the cervix, so the patient can be taught to make a vaginal inspection and can quickly ascertain the presence of the device. (See Figure 22.)

The method by which intra-uterine devices prevent pregnancy is not completely clear, but it seems that they interfere with implantation.

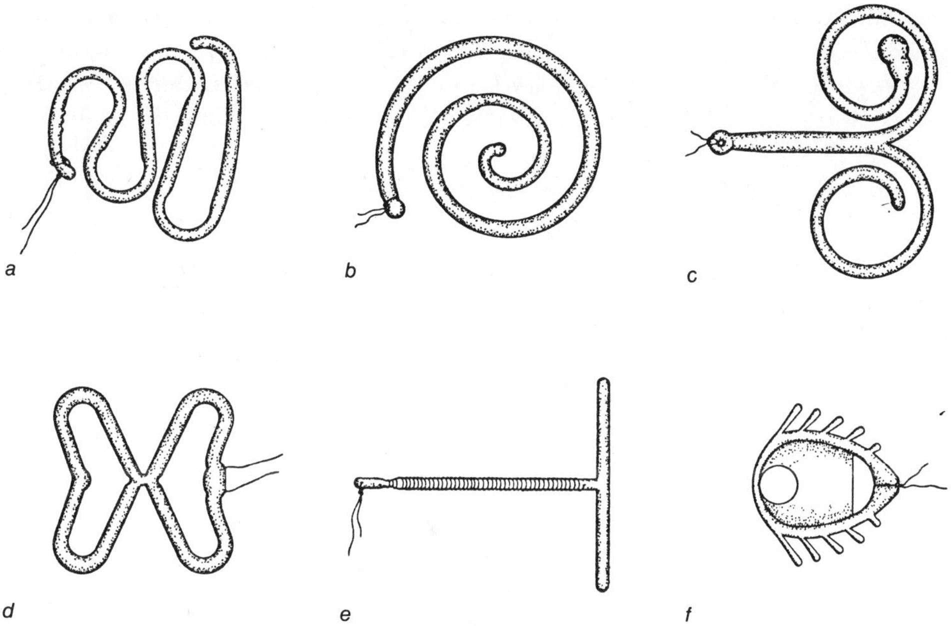

Figure 22. The intra-uterine devices shown are: a. the Lippes loop, b. the Margulies spiral, c. the double coil, d. the Birnberg bow, e. the copper T, f. the Dalkon shield.

The patient often experiences intermenstrual spotting, increased menstruation, and cramping during the first month or two the intra-uterine device is in place. After this she is unaware of its presence. Some women cannot use an IUCD because of expulsion, bleeding, or discomfort. The devices are not recommended for women who have not been pregnant because the uterus of nulliparas is too small and the cervical canal too narrow, thus causing severe pain and bleeding.

Intra-uterine devices are less effective than the pill. But unlike oral contraception, no continuous motivation is necessary.

Patients with IUCDs are given yearly appointments for follow-up visits. They are told to see their physician sooner in case they have any complaints, expel the device, or want to conceive again.

Diaphragm. Before oral contraceptives were developed, the safest and most frequently prescribed method was a combination of an occlusive vaginal diaphragm and a spermicidal jelly. It is necessary that the physician fit the diaphragm, instruct the patient in its use, and make certain, by having her return with the diaphragm in place after practicing its use at home, that she can insert it properly.

In order for the diaphragm to be effective, it must be combined with a spermicidal preparation that will immobilize and kill all sperm within about six hours following coitus. The spermicidal preparation may be applied either to the inside or the outside of the dome of the diaphragm and its rim. The diaphragm must be inserted before intercourse and left in place at least six hours after intercourse. It may be left inserted as long as 24 hours.

Although the diaphragm method offers a high level of protection, occasional failures may be expected because of improper insertion or displacement during sex relations.

The diaphragm should be refitted every two years and after each pregnancy.

Spermicidal jellies, foams, and tablets. These are chemical products inserted into the vagina before intercourse. Their purpose is to coat the vaginal wall and cervix, thereby exposing the sperm to their destructive action. They possibly act as a mechanical barrier as well.

The spermicidal preparations alone offer less protection than a combination of the spermicidal jelly and a diaphragm. The vaginal foams appear to be most effective; the tablets are the least effective because they may fail to melt after they have been placed in the vagina.

Rhythm. The human ovum probably survives no longer than 48 hours after it has been extruded from the ovary, and the life of the ejaculated sperm is little, if at all, longer. If coitus is avoided during the fertile period (three to four days before and after ovulation), unprotected intercourse during the safe period (the other days of the cycle) should not produce a pregnancy. Ovulation occurs fairly regularly about 14 days before the onset of menstruation, and the safe period can be calculated reasonably accurately in women whose cycles vary by no more than a day or two. Variations in the length of the menstrual cycles are ordinarily due to differences in the length of the preovulatory rather than the postovulatory phase; therefore, in women with grossly irregular cycles the fertile period can be calculated only in retrospect. Basal temperature curves will indicate the time of ovulation, but they are not satisfactory as a means of contraception because the temperature rise follows rather than precedes the rupture of the follicle.

If a patient with a regular cycle will avoid intercourse for three or four days before and after the calculated day of ovulation she will not become pregnant unless she occasionally ovulates at an unusual time. Use of the safe period with its relatively narrow margin of safety is quite satisfactory for people who want more children, but it is not certain enough for those in whom pregnancy must for one reason or another be avoided.

Surgical Methods of Birth Control

Hysterectomy. Hysterectomy, or removal of the uterus, is the most drastic and surest means of sterilization. It is customarily used only in patients presenting a medical indication for it. Many patients desiring sterilization are patients with relaxed pelvic support secondary to previous childbirth. A vaginal hysterectomy and an anterior and posterior repair solve this problem. In the same way, patients with histories of metromenorrhagia, uterine fibroids, or endometriosis might also be treated satisfactorily by hysterectomy.

Sterilization at the time of repeat cesarean section might be accomplished by cesarean hysterectomy or tubal ligation. Cesarean hysterectomy is the more dangerous procedure from the standpoint of hemorrhage.

Aside from hysterectomy, other sterilization operations, usually irreversible, for men and women are based on the same strategy: cutting the tubes that carry the sex cells on their paths toward union and conception. In the female this involves the fallopian tubes. In the male it involves the vas deferens (literally the "carry-away vessel") which arises from each testicle to carry the spermatozoa to the prostate gland, from which they are transported in the seminal fluid for ejaculation through the urethra.

Tubal Ligation. In this procedure the fallopian tubes are tied and severed; most surgeons also remove part of each tube. As mentioned previously, tubal ligation is often done at the time a patient has her third or fourth cesarean section because the couple has decided that this will be her last pregnancy and because many physicians are of the opinion that more cesarean sections are unsafe for the mother.

The operation is also frequently performed on women who have just given birth to babies normally. Within 36 hours after the delivery, the surgeon makes a three- or four-inch incision in the mother's lower abdomen to reach the tubes. Physicians prefer to do this type of surgery in the immediate postpartum period because this ensures that they are not interfering with an unknown pregnancy.

Laparoscopy. In recent years gynecologists have been seeking a means of reaching and severing the fallopian tubes without making a long pelvic incision. They have succeeded with the aid of the laparoscope, a tube containing at its end a light less than half an inch in diameter. Two incisions less than one half inch long are made just below the umbilicus (see Figure 23).

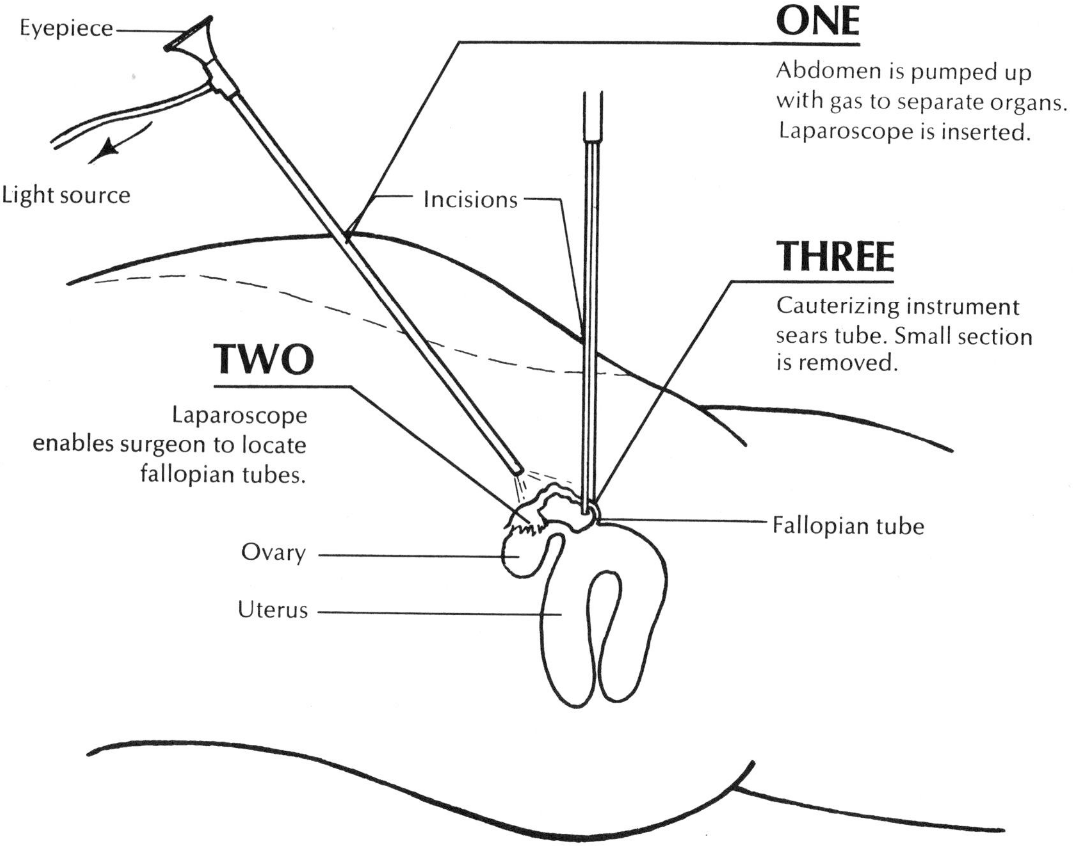

Figure 23. Laparoscopy. (© 1973 by Medical Economics Company. Reprinted with permission from *RN Magazine, 36:*4, April 1973.)

Through one, after blowing in carbon dioxide to separate the organs, the physician inserts the electric cautery and a tiny surgical knife. The operation, under general anesthesia, takes about 30 minutes, and the patient may leave the hospital within 24 hours.

The simplest development in sterilization of women, requiring only local anesthesia, is reported by a physician from New York. He has special instruments that enable him to operate through an incision slightly more than one inch long in the vaginal wall; he is able to reach and tie off both tubes in about ten minutes. This vaginal approach leaves the patient with no visible scars, and she can go home in 24 to 48 hours after the operation.

Ovariotexy. Two Australian gynecologists have devised a reversible sterilization procedure for women. It consists of wrapping the ovaries in a silastic bag and burying them beneath the peritoneum. Thus they are removed from the vicinity of the fallopian tubes and are unavailable to sperms. The use of the silastic bag adds an advantage to burying the ovary beneath the peritoneum in that another barrier is placed between the ovary and adjacent connective tissue. The name of the procedure, ovariotexy, is derived from the Greek word *texy,* which means woven and refers to the bag.

No postoperative complication occurred in any of the patients, and after periods of two months to one year none had complaints and none were pregnant. Pelvic examination revealed no ovarian swelling or any other abnormality.

Vasectomy. This sterilization procedure for the male corresponds to tubal ligation in the female. After injecting a local anesthetic, the surgeon makes an incision about half an inch long on one side of the scrotum, draws out one vas, and cuts out a section up to one inch long. He usually cauterizes the remaining stumps of the vas and ties them with nonabsorbable thread. The surgeon then sutures the small wound and repeats the procedure on the other side.

The vasectomy patient undergoes no hormonal changes; neither does his female counterpart following tubal ligation. He continues to form sperms which stay in the testicles and are reabsorbed. Eventually his body manufactures fewer of them. However, some sperms are left past the vas deferens at the time of the operation, so for the first month the patient is advised to use contraceptive precautions during intercourse. Most surgeons require that their patients return after four to twelve months and leave a semen sample for analysis to make sure that neither vas deferens has joined itself together again.

Reversible Male Sterilization. Two methods of reversible male sterilization appear feasible and are now being researched. One is a small tantalum clamp which is applied to the vas deferens with sufficient pressure to occlude it but not to cause atrophy or scarring. When the clamp is removed, fertility is restored. This clamp is now being used experimentally in India.

Work is also being done on a fluid plastic which is injected into the vas deferens and followed by a hardening agent to create a rubber plug in the vas. In extensive experiments it was found that this lasts for only about one year. In that time the spermatic juices are able to dissolve the plug, so better materials must still be found. Restoring fertility seems to pose no problem; a small incision over the vas allows the rubber plug to be removed.

The latest experiment, done at Johns Hopkins University, involves the injection of certain chemical compounds which act as sclerosing agents. The principal advantage of this method lies in the speed with which it can be performed—a mere two minutes instead of the usual one half hour for the conventional vasectomy. Other advantages are that the procedure is painless, carries little risk of infection or hematoma, and requires no surgical facilities. Furthermore, it eliminates the use of the scalpel, which to some men suggests castration. There is about a 50 per cent chance of reversibility.

FAMILY PLANNING PROGRAMS

The private patient has her own physician available for counseling on birth control matters. For patients attending clinic facilities various health agencies provide family planning services to women desiring it. Among these facilities are those operated by Planned Parenthood, city or state board of health departments, tax-supported and voluntary hospitals, and public health departments. Many of these agencies are funded by federal grants earmarked for family planning services by the U.S. Department of Health, Education and Welfare.

It is wise to inquire about the facilities in your own community from your instructor, supervisor, or local health department in order to assist patients needing this information.

FAMILY PLANNING REVIEWED

1. Identify the different methods of conception control described below.

The practice of temporary abstinence from sexual relations during the fertile period: (a) ______________________________

A device that, when properly placed in the vagina, covers the cervical os and holds a spermicidal preparation against the cervix: (b) ______________

A hormonal preparation that functions to prevent pregnancy by inhibiting ovulation: (c) ______________________________

A preparation that is applied within the vagina and is capable of immobilizing and killing spermatozoa and blocking the cervical os: (d) __________

A device, usually plastic, that is inserted into the uterus: (e) ______________

2. List the methods of nonsurgical conception control in order of effectiveness, beginning with the one having the lowest failure rate when it is in constant use:

(a)

(b)

(c)

(d)

(e)

You are reviewing with Mrs. Irene Fuller the instructions which her doctor gave her for taking contraceptive pills.

3. Circle the days on the calendar (Figure 24) when Mrs. Fuller should take the oral contraceptive. (The underlined days indicate menstruation.)

4. Mrs. Fuller asks you what she should do in case she does not menstruate after a course of the pills. What do you answer?

5. If you advise her to resume taking the pills, mark an "X" through the day on which she must restart taking the pills.

6. How frequently is the oral contraceptive taken?

			1	2	3	4
5	6	7	8	9	10	11
12	13	14	15	16	17	18
19	20	21	22	23	24	25
26	27	28	29	30	1	2
3	4	5	6	7	8	9
10	11	12	13	14	15	16
17	18	19	20	21	22	23
24	25	26	27	28	29	30
31						

Figure 24.

7. What is the action of spermicidal preparations?

8. Where should the spermicidal preparation be placed (by means of an applicator) when used as the sole means of contraception?

9. When properly positioned, a diaphragm covers the ______________

____.

10. For best results a diaphragm should be used in conjunction with ___

____.

11. What time of the menstrual cycle is safest for the insertion of an intra-uterine device? Why?

12. Name the side effects which may occur following the insertion of an intra-uterine device.

13. What do you advise a patient who tells you over the phone that she believes she expelled her IUCD?

14. What event(s) does each of the methods listed below block or otherwise interrupt so as to prevent pregnancy?

(a) Diaphragm method: ______________________________

(b) Intra-uterine devices: ______________________________

(c) Oral contraceptives: ______________________________

(d) Spermicidal preparations: ______________________________

Refer to the basal body temperature chart (Figure 25) while reviewing with Mrs. Ann Gibbs the rhythm method.

15. What was the temperature just prior to ovulation?

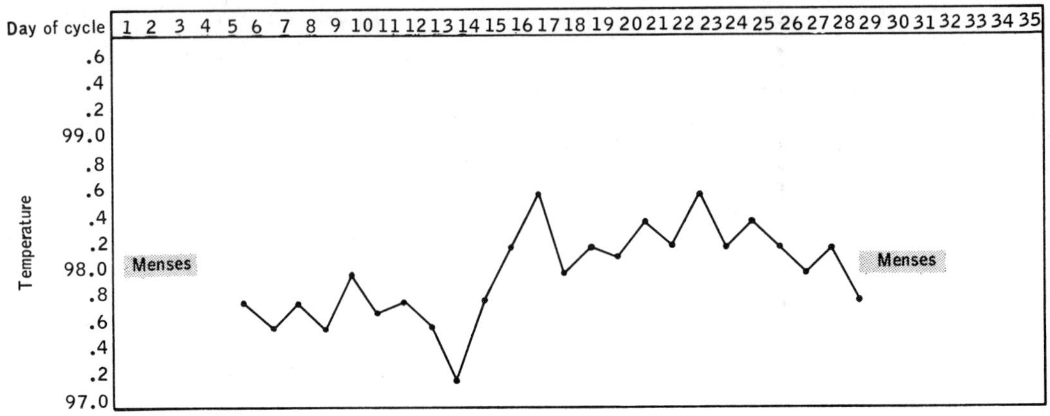

Figure 25. Basal Body Temperature During the Menstrual Cycle

16. When did ovulation occur?

17. The period of ovulation is characterized by:

☐ (a) A temperature drop followed by a temperature rise

☐ (b) A temperature rise followed by a temperature drop

18. You point out the fertile period to Mrs. Gibbs. On the chart this is the period from day __________ to day __________.

19. When using the rhythm period, what precaution should be taken during the fertile period?

20. Explain why a patient should, before using the rhythm method, keep careful records of the lengths of her menstrual cycles for at least eight months and preferably for one year.

21. Name the facilities available in your community where women can obtain help in family planning.

22. State your own attitude toward family planning.

23. Discuss the extent of counseling which your position toward family planning allows you.

REVIEW QUESTIONS

Circle the correct or best answer.

1. The ultimate goal of maternity care is:
   a. Safe care of mother and baby during the maternity cycle.
   b. A liveborn baby.
   c. Provision for total care of the entire family.
   d. Early medical supervision.

2. Statistics show that in our society:
   a. Marriages are occurring in younger age groups.
   b. Most couples are adequately prepared for marriage and a family.
   c. Marriages are occurring across cultural, social, and religious backgrounds.
   d. Marriages in the older age group (20 to 30 years) are on the upswing.
      (1) d is correct.
      (2) a, b, and c are correct.
      (3) a and c are correct.
      (4) All are correct.

3. During the last quarter of the twentieth century we will be faced with:
   a. An increasing number of women of childbearing age.
   b. The demand of the public at large to have a say in the delivery of maternity care.
   c. The possibility of achieving zero population growth.
   d. The popularity of the nurse-midwife and the maternity nursing specialist in providing obstetric care.
      (1) a is correct.
      (2) a and d are correct.
      (3) a, b, and c are correct.
      (4) All are correct.

4. The vaginal canal normally has:
   a. An acid environment.
   b. An alkaline environment.
   c. A neutral environment.
   d. An environment difficult to determine.

5. The internal genitalia in the female are the:
   a. Uterus, fallopian tubes, and ovaries.
   b. Uterus, vagina, and ovaries.
   c. Uterus, labia majora, and clitoris.
   d. Ovaries, uterus, and Bartholin's glands.

6. The adult bony pelvis is made up of:
   a. 2 bones.
   b. 4 bones.
   c. 6 bones.
   d. 8 bones.

7. The female pelvis differs from the male pelvis in that:
   a. It is heavier in construction.
   b. It is lighter in construction.
   c. It is deeper and narrower.
   d. The pubic arch is narrower.

8. The primordial follicles are usually found in the:
   a. Ovary.
   b. Fallopian tubes.
   c. Uterus.
   d. Cervix.

9. The hormones responsible for the menstrual cycle are:
   a. Estrogen and progesterone.
   b. Gonadotrophins.
   c. Gonadotrophins and estrogen.
   d. Gonadotrophins, estrogen, and progesterone.

10. The hormone(s) responsible for maturation of the graafian follicle is (are):
    a. Follicle-stimulating hormone.
    b. Luteinizing hormone.
    c. Follicle-stimulating hormone and estrogen.
    d. Follicle-stimulating hormone and progesterone.

11. The ovaries:
    a. Produce the luteinizing hormone.
    b. Inhibit the production of the primordial follicle.
    c. Produce estrogen and progesterone which are responsible for the uterine changes occurring during the menstrual cycle.
    d. Produce hormones which are oxytocic in nature.

12. Ovulation may be defined as the:
    a. Maturation of the graafian follicle.
    b. Rupture of the graafian follicle.
    c. Seepage of blood through the vagina.
    d. Follicular phase of the menstrual cycle.

13. Ovulation:
    a. Occurs at the time of menstruation.
    b. Occurs approximately 14 days after the onset of menstruation.
    c. Occurs approximately 14 days before the onset of menstruation.
    d. Occurs in the middle of the menstrual cycle.

14. The time of ovulation may be determined by the taking of the basal temperature. The temperature:
   a. Drops at the time of ovulation.
   b. Drops and then rises at the time of ovulation.
   c. Drops, rises, and drops again at the time of ovulation.
   d. Remains constant throughout the menstrual cycle.

15. Maturation of the ovum and sperm is a process in which:
   a. There is an elevation of hormones in the blood.
   b. There is a division and reduction of chromosomes during oogenesis and spermatogenesis.
   c. Gonadotrophins from the anterior pituitary are inhibited.
   d. There is an increase in the number of chromosomes during oogenesis and spermatogenesis.

16. Fertilization normally occurs:
   a. In the fallopian tube.
   b. In the abdominal cavity.
   c. In the uterus.
   d. In the ovary.

17. Penetration of the chorionic villi into the maternal surface is called:
   a. Fertilization.
   b. Impregnation.
   c. Fecundation.
   d. Implantation.

18. Implantation normally occurs:
   a. On the anterior or posterior portion of the fundus.
   b. In the fallopian tube.
   c. In the lower uterine segment.
   d. In the abdominal cavity.

19. The placenta is distinctly formed by the end of the:
   a. First month of gestation.
   b. Third month of gestation.
   c. Fifth month of gestation.
   d. Seventh month of gestation.

20. The change which occurs in fetal circulation soon after birth is:
   a. Replacement of the ductus nevosus and hypogastric arteries by fibrous cords.
   b. Patency of the ductus arteriosus.
   c. Closing of the foramen ovale.
   d. Expansion of the lungs.

21. Amniotic fluid is believed to be derived from:
    a. The mother's blood.
    b. Fetal urine.
    c. The amniotic epithelium.
    d. Both mother and baby.
        (1) a only is correct.
        (2) a and b are correct.
        (3) a, b, and c are correct.
        (4) All are correct.

22. The placenta functions as:
    a. An intermediary organ supplying nourishment to the fetus and returning his waste substances.
    b. A gland producing hormones which benefit both mother and fetus.
    c. A barrier to prevent certain substances from entering the fetal circulation.
    d. All of the above.

23. Which of the following is not a property of the amniotic fluid:
    a. Its normal amount is from 700 to 2000 cc.
    b. It provides mechanical protection for the fetus.
    c. Its composition is acid.
    d. Its specific gravity is between 1.006 and 1.015.

24. At the end of the first trimester of pregnancy, there is (are):
    a. An increase in blood volume.
    b. A decrease in the stroke volume of the heart.
    c. An increase in diastolic blood pressure.
    d. All of the above.

25. Weight gain during pregnancy is approximately:
    a. 9 to 14 lbs.
    b. 12 to 17 lbs.
    c. 18 to 25 lbs.
    d. 26 to 32 lbs.

26. A pregnant woman usually needs ______ grams of protein daily.
    a. 45
    b. 60
    c. 90
    d. 120

27. Movements of the baby felt by the mother are known as:
    a. Lightening.
    b. Quickening.
    c. Engagement.
    d. Ballottement.

28. Fetal growth is most rapid during the:
    a. Implantation phase.
    b. First trimester.
    c. Second trimester.
    d. Third trimester.

29. Frequency of urination causes the pregnant woman some concern mainly:
    a. During the first trimester.
    b. During the second trimester.
    c. Following lightening.
    d. At the time of quickening.
        (1) a and c are correct.
        (2) b and d are correct.
        (3) a and d are correct.
        (4) b and d are correct.

30. Regarding which of the minor disorders of pregnancy would you advise the patient?
    a. Morning sickness
    b. Pernicious vomiting
    c. Edema
    d. Spotting

31. Which of the following foods is most nearly equivalent to 1 cup of whole milk as a source of protein and calcium?
    a. 2-inch cube of cheddar cheese
    b. ½ cup of cottage cheese
    c. 1 serving of ice cream
    d. ½ cup whipped cream

32. When supplementary iron is given the patient should be told to expect:
    a. Diarrhea.
    b. Black stools.
    c. Black stools and possible constipation.
    d. Heartburn.

33. Heartburn during pregnancy results from:
    a. Increased work load of the heart.
    b. Increased stomach acidity.
    c. Increased peristalsis.
    d. Decreased gastric motility with backflow of stomach contents into the esophagus.

34. Heartburn during pregnancy may be alleviated by:
    a. Decreased intake of carbohydrate.
    b. Increased intake of protein.
    c. Use of sodium bicarbonate.
    d. Use of aluminum hydroxide gel.

35. The fetal heartbeat can be heard with the stethoscope by the _____ week of gestation:
   a. Sixth
   b. Twelfth
   c. Twentieth
   d. Ninth

36. The placenta at term weighs:
   a. 1500-1600 gm.
   b. One-third of the weight of the fetus.
   c. 500-600 gm.
   d. 200-300 gm.

450 gm = 1 lb.

37. Constipation during pregnancy is best treated by:
   a. Regular use of laxatives such as milk of magnesia.
   b. Light exercise such as walking.
   c. Increased cellulose and fluids in the diet.
   d. Regular use of glycerine suppositories.

38. Which of the following would not be expected to relieve varicose veins in pregnancy?
   a. Resting with both feet elevated.
   b. Discontinuing use of round garters.
   c. Wearing a well-fitted bra.
   d. Using elastic stockings.

39. Which of the following does not apply to an ectopic pregnancy?
   a. It can occur in the ovary.
   b. It can occur in the uterine tube.
   c. It can occur in the uterus.
   d. It can occur in the abdominal cavity.

40. Natural childbirth classes prepare the woman to expect that:
   a. She will be able to handle the labor contractions if she does the breathing and relaxation exercises as taught.
   b. She will be coached by her husband and the nursing staff during labor.
   c. She may receive medication and some type of anesthesia, other than general.
   d. She will experience an unusually satisfying feeling of accomplishment when her baby is born.
      (1) a and d are correct.
      (2) b and d are correct.
      (3) b and c are correct.
      (4) All are correct.

41. The purpose of teaching exercises for childbirth is:
    a. To develop strong abdominal muscles.
    b. To teach relaxation and pushing techniques.
    c. To promote good posture.
    d. To teach various breathing techniques for use during labor, to explain comfortable positions, and to train certain muscle groups for the second stage of labor.

42. When you are explaining to the expectant mother the importance of reporting danger symptoms, which of the following should you teach her to report to the physician promptly?
    a. Constipation.
    b. Heartburn.
    c. Vaginal bleeding.
    d. Swelling of the face and hands.
    e. Swelling of the feet and legs which persists overnight.
    f. Backache.
    g. Blurring of vision.
    h. Morning sickness.
    i. Severe headache in the second half of pregnancy.
    j. Marked diminution in urinary output.
    k. Excessive salivation.
    l. Persistent abdominal pain or tenderness.
    m. Fever, with or without chills.
    n. Hemorrhoids.
    o. Rhythmic, painful uterine contractions occuring more frequently than every 10 minutes.
    p. Gush of clear fluid from the vagina.
    q. Muscular cramps.

Choose from Column II the definitions which most accurately define the terms in Column I.

Column I			Column II
43. Primigravida	....	a.	A woman in labor.
		b.	A woman pregnant for the first time.
44. Gravida	....	c.	A woman who has just given birth.
		d.	A pregnant woman.
45. Multipara	....	e.	A woman who has had two or more children.
46. Parturient	....		
47. Puerpera	....		

48. Legal abortions may be performed:
    a. Without a state's interference if they are doctor-approved and done within the first three months of pregnancy.
    b. Only in those states which have liberalized abortion laws.
    c. Only to preserve the mother's life.
    d. During the last trimester of pregnancy subject only to the husband's and wife's consent.

49. If active syphilis is not treated in a pregnant patient she may:
    a. Abort.
    b. Have a premature delivery.
    c. Bear a child having congenital syphilis.
    d. All of the above.

50. The treatment of choice for syphilis is:
    a. Sulfur compounds.
    b. Cortisone preparations.
    c. Penicillin products.
    d. Mono-amine oxidase inhibitors.

51. Gonorrhea exhibits the following characteristic:
    a. An individual may have the gonococcus and still be asymptomatic.
    b. The bacteria are air-borne.
    c. The bacteria can be transmitted through breaks or cuts in the skin.
    d. The bacteria can be transmitted to the fetus via the placenta.

52. Gonorrhea occurs most often among the:
    a. 25 to 35-year-old age group.
    b. 30 to 40-year-old age group.
    c. 15 to 25-year-old age group.
    d. None of the above.

53. Untreated gonorrhea may cause:
    a. Pelvic inflammatory disease.
    b. Sterility.
    c. Infection in unsuspecting contacts.
    d. Blindness in the baby following childbirth.
        (1) a and c are correct.
        (2) d is correct.
        (3) b and d are correct.
        (4) a, b, c, and d are correct.

54. Epidemic rubella contracted in the second trimester of pregnancy may cause:
    a. Stillbirth.
    b. Cataracts in the infant's eyes.
    c. The infant to have a low birth weight.
    d. None of the above.

55. In caring for the patient with hyperemesis gravidarum the nurse should:
    a. Maintain an accurate record of intake and output.
    b. Urge the patient to force down a regular diet.
    c. Be on the alert for acetone breath.
    d. Allow no visitors under any circumstances.
        (1) a, b, and c are correct.
        (2) a, c and d are correct.
        (3) a, b and d are correct.
        (4) a and c are correct.

Mrs. Watson, a 17-year-old primigravida, was admitted to the hospital during her thirty-second week of pregnancy, because the following symptoms were found during her prenatal visit: She had gained 10 pounds since her last visit three weeks ago; blood pressure was 168/98; urinalysis revealed a +2 albumin. In addition she had edema of the hands and feet. She stated that she had headaches. Her orders on admission include: absolute bedrest; 1200 calorie, low-salt, high-protein diet; checking of blood pressure, pulse, and fetal heart q 2 hrs.; phenobarbital gr. ½ q id; Diuril 0.5 gm. daily; weigh q A.M.; urinalysis for albumin q 4 hrs.; intake and output records. The diagnosis was pre-eclampsia.

Questions 56-60 apply to Mrs. Watson.

56. Bedrest is essential in pre-eclampsia, since it:
    a. Prevents eclampsia.
    b. Mobilizes tissue fluid, thereby lowering blood pressure.
    c. Improves circulation and decreases leg edema.
    d. Prevents premature labor and delivery.

57. Diuril, a diuretic, is effective in decreasing tissue fluid by:
    a. Preventing reabsorption of sodium and chlorides in the kidney tubules.
    b. Drawing tissue fluid into the bloodstream for elimination through the kidneys.
    c. Increasing urinary output.
    d. Acting as a hypertonic drug.

58. A low-salt, high-protein diet is ordered:
    a. To limit the carbohydrate intake.
    b. To prevent weight gain.
    c. To provide a low-fat intake.
    d. Because pre-eclampsia seems prevalent in women with poorly balanced low-protein diets.

59. Phenobarbital acts as a:
    a. Sedative.
    b. Hypnotic.
    c. Anti-hypertensive.
    d. Stimulant.

60. If Mrs. Watson's diagnosis had been eclampsia she would have shown which of the following symptoms:
   a. Concentrated, scant urine.
   b. Increased body temperature.
   c. Convulsion(s), with or without coma.
   d. Rise in blood pressure.
      (1) a and c are correct.
      (2) b and d are correct.
      (3) All are correct.
      (4) c is correct.

61. Which of the following are typical symptoms of abruptio placentae?
   a. Vaginal bleeding.
   b. Uterine tetany.
   c. Abdominal pain and tenderness.
   d. A chill followed by a temperature of 102°F. or higher.
      (1) a, b, and c are correct.
      (2) b, c, and d are correct.
      (3) a, b, and d are correct.
      (4) All are correct.

62. Which of the following is the most common cause of bleeding during the third trimester?
   a. Threatened abortion.
   b. Hydatid mole.
   c. Placenta previa.
   d. Ectopic pregnancy.

63. The number of diabetic women who become pregnant has:
   a. Markedly increased since the introduction of insulin.
   b. Decreased since the introduction of insulin.
   c. Remained the same since the introduction of insulin.
   d. Markedly decreased since the introduction of hypoglycemic drugs.

64. RhoGAM is administered within 72 hours after delivery:
   a. To all Rh-negative mothers.
   b. Only to sensitized Rh-negative mothers.
   c. To Rh-negative mothers, free of sensitization to the Rh factor, whose babies are Rh-positive.
   d. Only to Rh-negative mothers whose babies have a positive Coombs test.

65. The mother who has active tuberculosis should not nurse her baby:
   a. Because the infant may become infected by way of tubercle bacilli exhaled by his mother.
   b. Because the infant may become infected as a result of contamination of the milk.
   c. Because lactation is a drain on the mother's strength.
   d. Because nursing may cause the formation of a chancre on the mother's breast.

(1) a and b are correct.
(2) a and c are correct.
(3) b and d are correct.
(4) b and c are correct.

Choose from Column II the definitions which most accurately define the terms in Column I.

Column I

66. Fontanelle ....
67. Attitude ....
68. Presentation ....
69. Position ....
70. Engagement ....
71. Station ....
72. Lightening ....
73. Sutures ....
74. Molding ....
75. Bimanual ....

Column II

a. The shaping of the fetal head to adjust itself to the birth canal.
b. The membranous joints between the bones of the fetal skull.
c. The conformation of the fetal spine—flexed or extended.
d. The sensation of decreased abdominal distention produced by the descent of the presenting part into the pelvic cavity.
e. The widened area at the point where sutures meet.
f. The relationship of a predetermined point on the fetus to one of the four quadrants of the maternal pelvis.
g. The rebound of a fetal part when displaced by the examining finger either through the abdominal wall or the vagina.
h. The term used to describe the relationship of the baby's spine to the mother's spine.
i. The relationship of the presenting part to the ischial spines.
j. Listening to sounds produced by heart beats.
k. The descent of the greatest diameter of the presenting part to a level below the pelvic inlet.
l. Examination by both hands.

76. Among the reasons for the prevalence of unmarried motherhood is (are) the following:
   a. Women's dislike of "planned" sex.
   b. The feeling that "it can't happen to me" or "I thought I was in a safe period."
   c. Lack of knowledge about contraceptives, particularly among young girls.
   d. All of the above.

77. Today's unmarried pregnant women are more likely:
   a. To keep their babies and raise them themselves.
   b. To abandon their babies to their parents for care.
   c. To place their babies for adoption.
   d. To force the natural father to either support them financially or marry them.

78. The unmarried expectant mother tends:
   a. To be more candid about her pregnancy.
   b. To try to hide her pregnancy.
   c. To avoid seeking antepartal care.
   d. To spurn the natural father.

79. If the first day of a patient's last normal menstrual period was January 1, which of the following would be the correct FDC:
   a. October 1
   b. October 8
   c. November 8
   d. September 8

80. It is sometimes difficult to determine whether or not a patient is in true labor. True labor is distinguished from false labor in that:
   a. Contractions come at irregular intervals.
   b. The patient complains of pain, chiefly in the lower abdomen and groin.
   c. There is definite effacement and dilatation of the cervix.
   d. Contractions do not increase in severity, intensity, or duration.

81. Labor is divided into three stages. The first stage is:
   a. From the complete dilatation of the cervix to the delivery of the baby.
   b. From the onset of labor to the complete dilatation of the cervix.
   c. From the delivery of the baby to the expulsion of the secundines.
   d. From the expulsion of the secundines for one hour.

82. The frequency of uterine contractions is determined by timing:
   a. From the end of one contraction to the beginning of the next contraction.
   b. From the beginning of one contraction to the beginning of the next contraction.
   c. From the beginning of one contraction to the end of the next contraction.
   d. From the end of one contraction to the end of the next contraction.

83. The strength of a contraction is determined by palpating the uterus. A strong contraction is one in which:
   a. The uterine wall is firm but can be indented with the examining finger.
   b. The uterine wall becomes hard and cannot be indented by the examining finger.
   c. The uterine wall stays firm from one contraction to the next.
   d. None of the above.

84. Uterine contractions during labor are:
   a. Rhythmical but not equally strong.
   b. All of the same frequency.
   c. All of the same duration.
   d. All equally strong.

85. When admitting an obstetric patient in early labor to the labor room, the first thing to do is to see that:
   a. The perineal shave is done immediately.
   b. The clothes are checked.
   c. Good rapport is established with the patient.
   d. Temperature, pulse, respiration, blood pressure, and fetal heart tone are taken.

86. The patient should be instructed to bear down with her contractions:
   a. During the last part of the first stage of labor.
   b. At the beginning of the second stage of labor.
   c. During the latter part of the second stage.
   d. Whenever she feels the desire to bear down with her contractions.

87. It is important that an admission temperature, pulse, and respiration be taken on all patients admitted in labor:
   a. Because it is a hospital routine.
   b. Because an elevated temperature may indicate infection.
   c. Because the patient expects it.
   d. None of the above.

88. The patient in labor should be encouraged to void:
   a. Because a full bladder may hinder labor by preventing the presenting part from descending.
   b. Because several urine specimens are required during labor.
   c. To prevent the need to have the patient catheterized at the time of delivery.
   d. To test the urine for spillage of acetone or albumin.

89. As a general rule, solid foods are withheld during labor because:
   a. The emptying time of the stomach is markedly prolonged during labor.
   b. There is danger that solid particles of food might be aspirated following the vomiting which sometimes occurs after the administration of certain medications, because of strong labor contractions, or during or following anesthesia.
   c. The emptying time of the stomach is not changed during labor.
   d. Normal labor is short enough so that a patient will suffer no actual harm if food is withheld.
      (1) a, b, and d are correct.
      (2) b, c, and d are correct.
      (3) a and b are correct.
      (4) b and d are correct.

90. Delivery is imminent in the multipara when:
   a. The contractions are coming every 2 to 3 minutes and are lasting 40 to 50 seconds.
   b. The membranes rupture.
   c. The cervix is completely dilated.
   d. Bloody show is present.

91. Medications commonly are given during the first stage of labor to:
   a. Dull the perception of pain.
   b. Produce a painless labor for the fetus.
   c. Keep the labor rooms quiet.
   d. Suppress oral, nasal, tracheal, and bronchial secretions.
      (1) a, b, and c are correct.
      (2) a, c, and d are correct.
      (3) b, c, and d are correct.
      (4) a and d are correct.

92. A factor which aids in the reduction of the need for large doses of medication during labor is:
   a. Antepartum teaching.
   b. The ability to control breathing.
   c. The presence of an understanding and interested person.
   d. Skilled nursing care.

93. Before delivery, a thorough cleansing of the vulva is carried out:
   a. To reduce the possibility of introducing contaminated material into the vagina.
   b. To sterilize the area around the birth canal.
   c. As a routine procedure.
   d. To refresh the patient.

94. An episiotomy is usually done:
   a. On a primigravida, because she always has a rigid perineum.
   b. On a multipara who has a relaxed perineum.
   c. On any patient in whom it appears that there will be a laceration of the perineum.
   d. Routinely on all patients.

95. A chill at the end of the third stage of labor usually indicates that:
   a. The patient is developing sepsis.
   b. The patient is having a nervous reaction to delivery.
   c. There is an intra-uterine hemorrhage.
   d. The patient has a high fever.

96. Labor usually progresses normally without complication, but the nurse must be constantly on the alert for any signs of impending danger. Some of these signs are:
   a. Meconium–stained amniotic fluid when the breech is presenting.
   b. Meconium–stained amniotic fluid when the vertex is presenting.
   c. Contractions which last more than 90 seconds.
   d. Fetal heart rate below 100.
      (1) a, c, and d are correct.
      (2) b, c, and d are correct.
      (3) c and d are correct.
      (4) b and d are correct.

97. In resuscitating the newborn infant, the following precautions should be observed:
   a. Gentle handling of the infant.
   b. Keeping the infant warm.
   c. Clearing the air passages.
   d. Having all necessary resuscitation equipment readily available for all deliveries.
      (1) a, b, and c are correct.
      (2) a, c, and d are correct.
      (3) b, c, and d are correct.
      (4) a, b, c, and d are correct.

98. In the case of an impending precipitate delivery the nurse should:
   a. Hold the head of the fetus back until the physician arrives.
   b. Give the patient ether.
   c. Remain with the patient, coach and assist her.
   d. Call the physician.

99. The patient who is watched closely seldom delivers before the personnel are ready for the delivery. In addition to cervical dilatation, which of the following symptoms should warn the nurse that the patient is approaching the end of the first stage of labor?
    a. A decrease in the strength of the contractions.
    b. The patient asks for the bedpan (to urinate).
    c. Nausea and vomiting.
    d. Rupture of the membranes following a strong contraction.
        (1) a, b, and c are correct.
        (2) a, c, and d are correct.
        (3) b, c, and d are correct.
        (4) None are correct.

100. Following delivery, the newborn infant should be:
    a. Kept warm.
    b. Observed closely for cyanosis.
    c. Observed closely for bleeding from the cord.
    d. Placed on his side to facilitate the drainage of mucus from the mouth.
        (1) a, b, c, and d are correct.
        (2) a, b, and c are correct.
        (3) a, b, and d are correct.
        (4) b and d are correct.

101. Low forceps delivery refers to the application of the forceps:
    a. To the head after it has entered the cavity of the pelvis.
    b. To the head after it has reached the perineum.
    c. To the head before it has entered the inlet.
    d. To the after-coming head in a breech extraction.

102. Frank breech is defined as:
    a. The position when the normal attitude of flexion is maintained and the fetus sits tailor-fashion on the pelvis.
    b. The position when one foot presents at the cervix.
    c. The position when the knees are extended, the thighs are flexed, and the breech alone presents.
    d. The position when both feet present at the cervix.

103. The low cervical cesarean section is the procedure of choice in many cases. When it is used:
    a. The incision is made in the contractile portion of the uterus.
    b. The incision is made in the lowermost portion of the uterus.
    c. The uterus is removed following the delivery of the baby.
    d. The incision is made extraperitoneally.

104. The most common indication for a cesarean section is:
a. Twins.
b. Breech presentation.
c. Previous cesarean section.
d. Prolonged labor.

105. Toxemia of pregnancy is not resolved until:
a. The urine is negative for albumin.
b. The blood pressure is normal.
c. The baby is delivered.
d. Convulsions have been ruled out.

106. Medical induction of labor consists of:
a. Administering a pain-relieving drug.
b. Rupturing the membranes.
c. Giving an oxytocic medication.
d. Cesarean section.

107. Dystocia refers to:
a. Fracture of the scapula of delivered infant.
b. Nerve injury to one side of baby's face.
c. Prolonged or difficult labor.
d. Precipitate delivery.

108. Among the causes for uterine inertia are:
a. Multiple pregnancy.
b. Hydramnios.
c. Presence of uterine fibroids.
d. Elderly primigravida.
(1) a and d are correct.
(2) c and d are correct.
(3) a and b are correct.
(4) a, b, c, and d are correct.

109. Medical indications for the induction of labor are:
a. Toxemia.
b. Diabetes.
c. Marginal placenta previa.
d. Membranes which are ruptured 12 to 24 hours prior to the onset of labor.
(1) b, c, and d are correct.
(2) a and b are correct.
(3) a, c, and d are correct.
(4) a, b, c, and d are correct.

110. In placenta accreta all or a portion of the placenta is abnormally adherent to the uterus because of previous damage to the endometrium. This may be caused by:
   a. Infected abortion.
   b. Repeated curettages.
   c. Uterine tumors.
   d. Radium radiation.
      (1) a and c are correct.
      (2) b, c, and d are correct.
      (3) c and d are correct.
      (4) a, b, c, and d are correct.

111. Treatment for placenta accreta may involve:
   a. Hysterectomy.
   b. Leaving the placenta in the uterus.
   c. Dilatation and curettage.
   d. Removal of the placenta by suction.
      (1) a and b are correct.
      (2) c and d are correct.
      (3) a, c, and d are correct.
      (4) a, b, c, and d are correct.

112. A second degree laceration of the perineum involves:
   a. The anterior margin of the perineum and the fourchette.
   b. The perineal body.
   c. The sphincter and muscle.
   d. None of the above.

113. The puerperium is that period:
   a. Which ends when menstruation is reestablished.
   b. Which lasts from the time of delivery to the establishment of lactation.
   c. Between the end of the third stage of labor and the essentially complete involution and healing of the pelvic structures.
   d. Which lies between childbirth and the mother's return home from the hospital.

114. Immediately after delivery the uterus should be:
   a. Well contracted with its upper border not above the level of the umbilicus.
   b. Well contracted with its upper border 3 to 4 fingerbreadths above the umbilicus.
   c. Relaxed with its upper border level with the umbilicus.
   d. Relaxed with its upper border 2 to 3 fingerbreadths below the umbilicus.

115. The watery, yellowish fluid secreted from the breasts before the milk comes in is called:
   a. Lochia.
   b. Engorgement.
   c. Colostrum.
   d. Ophthalmia neonatorum.

116. The secretion of milk from the delivered mother's breasts starts:
   a. Between the third and fourth day postpartum.
   b. Within 48 hours after delivery.
   c. Immediately following delivery.
   d. Between the sixth and eighth day postpartum.

117. Between the second and fourth day postpartum breast engorgement may occur. In the non-nursing mother the following steps may be beneficial:
   a. Pump the breasts.
   b. Apply ice bags to the breasts.
   c. Support the breasts with a snug-fitting breastbinder.
   d. Apply heat to the breasts.
      (1) a and d are correct.
      (2) b and c are correct.
      (3) a, b, and c are correct.
      (4) a, c, and d are correct.

118. After-pains are experienced:
   a. When the uterine muscles alternately relax and contract.
   b. By the primipara.
   c. By the multipara.
   d. The first three to four days postpartum.
      (1) b and d are correct.
      (2) a and c are correct.
      (3) a, c, and d are correct.
      (4) a, b, and d are correct.

119. The postpartum uterus must be watched very closely because of the danger of postpartum hemorrhage. The patient most likely to have it is:
   a. A primipara.
   b. A multipara.
   c. A woman who has just delivered twins.
   d. A woman who has just delivered a low-birth-weight infant.

120. The lochia is an indicator of the rate of healing of the uterus. In which succession does it appear?
   a. Alba, rubra, serosa.
   b. Rubra, alba, serosa.
   c. Rubra, serosa, alba.
   d. Serosa, rubra, alba.

121. Involution occurs most rapidly in:
   a. The primipara.
   b. The multipara.
   c. The mother who nurses her baby.
   d. The mother who ambulates early.

122. Frequently the newly delivered mother is unable to empty her bladder completely. Which of the following symptoms would cause the nurse to suspect that there may be residual urine?
   a. Displacement of the uterus upward.
   b. Frequency of urination.
   c. Lower abdominal pain.
   d. Edema of the perineum.
      (1) a, b, and c are correct.
      (2) b, c, and d are correct.
      (3) a, c, and d are correct.
      (4) a, b, c, and d are correct.

123. Factors which may contribute to sore and cracked nipples are:
   a. The antepartum use of "hardening" preparations.
   b. Nursing a very vigorous baby.
   c. Allowing the baby to nurse for long periods (half an hour or longer).
   d. Allowing the baby to grasp only the nipple itself while nursing.
      (1) a, b, c, and d are correct.
      (2) a, b, and c are correct.
      (3) a, c, and d are correct.
      (4) b, c, and d are correct.

124. Lactation is stimulated:
   a. By waiting until the "milk comes in" to take the baby to breast.
   b. By emptying the breasts.
   c. By applying ice bags to the breasts between feedings.
   d. By administering Deladumone at the beginning of the second stage of labor (at some hospitals it is given after delivery).

125. To the mother unfamiliar with what to expect of her baby, the nurse should explain that the following are normal in a newborn:
   a. Hiccoughing.
   b. Sneezing.
   c. Slight jaundice which appears about the third day.
   d. Startling movements when his crib is jarred.
      (1) a, b, and c are correct.
      (2) b and d are correct.
      (3) a, b, c, and d are correct.
      (4) a, c, and d are correct.

126. The newborn infant's needs can usually best be met by:
  a. The 4-hour schedule of feeding.
  b. The 3-hour schedule of feeding.
  c. The self-demand schedule of feeding.
  d. The 2-hour schedule of feeding.

127. Rooming-in is a plan whereby the baby is cared for at his mother's bedside. Which of the following statements is correct?
  a. All mothers should have their babies at their bedsides so that they may learn the technique of infant care.
  b. The rooming-in plan definitely reduces the number of professional personnel needed.
  c. The rooming-in plan should be flexible so that if a mother does not wish her baby at her bedside the baby may be placed in the nursery.
  d. A baby who has been at his mother's bedside should never be returned to the nursery because of the danger of infection to the other babies.

128. During the puerperium the first sign of infection is most frequently detected by an increase in:
  a. Temperature.
  b. Pulse rate.
  c. Lochial discharge.
  d. Blood pressure.

129. If treatment for sore and cracked nipples is not instituted the patient will probably develop:
  a. Caked breasts.
  b. Engorged breasts.
  c. Mastitis.
  d. Breast abscess.

130. Which of the following is not a symptom of localized pelvic infection?
  a. Fever.
  b. Rapid pulse.
  c. Pain and tenderness in the pelvic region.
  d. Normal lochia.

Choose from Column II the definitions which most accurately define the terms in Column I.

Column I		Column II
131. Parametritis.	....	a. Inflammation of the lining of the uterus.
132. Phlebitis.	....	b. A morbid condition due to pathogenic bacteria in the blood stream.

133. Phlegmasia alba dolens. ....

134. Puerperal sepsis. ....

135. Thrombophlebitis. ....

136. Mastitis. ....

137. Endometritis. ....

138. Septicemia. ....

c. An infection during the puerperium arising in the pelvic organs.

d. Phlebitis of the femoral vein with swelling and paleness of the leg.

e. Inflammation of the tissues around the uterus.

f. Inflammation of the mammary gland.

g. Inflammation of a vein.

h. Thrombosis combined with inflammation of a vein or veins.

139. Which of the following drug groups is not used in the treatment of puerperal infection?
   a. Sulfa drugs.
   b. Antibiotics.
   c. Oxytocics.
   d. Anticoagulants.

140. Of the methods of conception control listed, which gives virtually 100 per cent effectiveness?
   a. Intrauterine devices.
   b. Diaphragm.
   c. Oral contraceptives.
   d. Coitus interruptus.

141. Which of the following contraceptives requires consultation with a physician?
   a. Coitus interruptus.
   b. Vaginal foams.
   c. Diaphragm.
   d. Condom.

142. Some women who try intrauterine devices cannot use them satisfactorily because of:
   a. Expulsion.
   b. Bleeding.
   c. Discomfort.
   d. All of the above.

143. The use of effective contraceptives leads to:
   a. Population growth control.
   b. Reduced anxiety over unwanted pregnancy.
   c. Family planning.
   d. All of the above.

144. Of the surgical methods of birth control listed, which one is definitely irreversible?
   a. Vasectomy.
   b. Laparoscopy.
   c. Hysterectomy.
   d. Tubal ligation.

145. The primary focus of immediate care of the newborn is to:
   a. Do an Apgar scoring.
   b. Suction mucus to provide an open airway.
   c. Appraise the infant.
   d. Provide warmth.

146. Silver nitrate 1 per cent is instilled into the newborn's eyes to:
   a. Prevent staphylococcal infection.
   b. Prevent spirochetal infection.
   c. Prevent gonococcal infection.
   d. Prevent streptococcal infection.

147. The Apgar scoring is done to:
   a. Appraise the infant for birth defects.
   b. Appraise the infant for respiratory status.
   c. Appraise the infant for Rh sensitization.
   d. Appraise the infant for neurological development.

148. The daily caloric requirement of the newborn is:
   a. 15 to 25 calories per pound body weight.
   b. 25 to 30 calories per pound body weight.
   c. 35 to 40 calories per pound body weight.
   d. 45 to 50 calories per pound body weight.

149. The CHO content for the newborn is:
   a. 1/5 of total caloric requirement.
   b. 1/4 of total caloric requirement.
   c. 1/2 of total caloric requirement.
   d. 3/4 of total caloric requirement.

150. Which of the following statements are correct in considering psychological growth of the newborn?
   a. The infant's need for contact with a mother figure is greater than his need for food.
   b. The infant perceives the outside world by gratification as his needs are met.
   c. The cry is the infant's only defense mechanism.
   d. The interaction between mother and infant begins from the moment of conception.
      (1) a and c are correct.
      (2) b and c are correct.
      (3) b, c, and d are correct.
      (4) a, b, c, and d are correct.

151. Normal respirations in the newborn are:
- a. Regular, mostly initiated by the chest wall, 40 to 60 per minute.
- b. Irregular, abdominal, 30 to 40 per minute.
- c. Regular, abdominal, 60 to 80 per minute.
- d. Irregular, mostly initiated by the chest wall, 30 to 40 per minute.

152. Which of the following statements are correct?
- a. Rh sensitization causes physiologic jaundice of the newborn.
- b. The newborn with Rh problems is transfused with Rh-positive blood.
- c. The normal cord bilirubin is 2.5 to 3 mg. in 100 ml. or less.
- d. The Coombs test and amniotic fluid evaluation of the mother are used in determining antibody formation.
  - (1) a and c are correct.
  - (2) a, b, and c are correct.
  - (3) c and d are correct.
  - (4) a, b, c, and d are correct.

153. Which of the following relates to treatment and prevention of Rh sensitization?
- a. Phototherapy has been found effective in treating mild to moderately sensitized newborns.
- b. Intra-uterine transfusion may be the treatment of choice in severe to critical sensitization.
- c. RhoGAM is given to all Rh-negative mothers following delivery or abortion.
- d. RhoGAM provides an active immunity in the mother.
  - (1) b, c, and d are correct.
  - (2) a and c are correct.
  - (3) a and b are correct.
  - (4) a, b, c, and d are correct.

154. Which of the following statements relating to the newborn are correct?
- a. Cyanosis of hands and feet is common during the first 24 hours.
- b. Absence of grasp, Moro, and sucking reflexes indicates brain damage.
- c. Tremors, restlessness, irritability and a shrill cry indicate central nervous system damage.
- d. Milia are undeveloped sebaceous glands.
  - (1) a and b are correct.
  - (2) a and c are correct.
  - (3) a, b, and d are correct.
  - (4) a, b, c, and d are correct.

155. The infant receiving breast milk will most likely:
   a. Acquire immunity from antibodies received in feeding.
   b. Have a frequent and softer stool.
   c. Need to be fed more often since stomach empties sooner.
   d. Be free of allergies.
      (1) a is correct.
      (2) b and c are correct.
      (3) a and d are correct.
      (4) a, b, c, and d are correct.

156. The following characteristics are normal in newborns:
   a. A receding chin, rooting reflex.
   b. A skin erythema.
   c. Mongolian spots, milia.
   d. Head circumference larger than chest.
      (1) a is correct.
      (2) b and c are correct.
      (3) a and c are correct.
      (4) c and d are correct.

157. In the conduct of a premature labor and delivery:
   a. The use of analgesics and sedatives should be reduced to a minimum.
   b. Ether anesthesia should be used at the time of delivery.
   c. Low forceps should never be resorted to because the baby is so small.
   d. Episiotomy is rarely indicated.

158. In feeding the small premature infant:
   a. A soft, average-size nipple is usually satisfactory.
   b. Gavage feeding has been found most satisfactory since it reduces fatigue.
   c. The medicine dropper is the most satisfactory method since it eliminates fatigue.
   d. The technique of feeding is not important.

159. A low-birth-weight infant:
   a. Weighs more than 2500 gm.
   b. Weighs more than 3000 gm.
   c. Weighs less than 2500 gm.
   d. None of the above.

160. The leading cause of neonatal deaths in the United States is:
   a. The respiratory distress syndrome.
   b. Congenital malformations.
   c. Prematurity.
   d. Infections.

161. The low-birth-weight infant:
   a. Has a strong sucking reflex.
   b. Has an abundance of subcutaneous fat.
   c. Usually has an elevated temperature.
   d. Reflexes such as the grasp, Moro, etc. are not fully developed.

162. In gavaging a low-birth-weight infant:
   a. The standard length of tubing is inserted through the nose or mouth.
   b. Observation of respiration during the feeding is paramount.
   c. The gavage feedings are terminated upon the first indication of the infant's ability to suck.
   d. None of the above.

163. The care of the low-birth-weight infant by the parents:
   a. Should be initiated early and not just prior to discharge.
   b. Should be initiated at the time of discharge.
   c. Should be initiated when the nurse comes to visit the home following the baby's discharge.
   d. None of the above.

164. Which of the following statements is true?
   a. The bacteria causing syphilis are too large to cross the placenta.
   b. Treatment of syphilis early in pregnancy does not reduce the risk of the disease in the newborn.
   c. Untreated spirochetal infection is responsible for congenital syphilis in the newborn.
   d. None of the above.

165. Caput succedaneum is:
   a. A circumscribed area of edema formed on the fetal head during labor.
   b. Jaundice sometimes seen in the normal newborn infant.
   c. An accumulation of blood under the periosteum, especially of the parietal bones, following labor.
   d. A hemorrhage occuring within the cranium.

166. A cephalhematoma may be defined as:
   a. A circumscribed area of edema formed on the fetal head during labor.
   b. A hemorrhage occurring within the cranium.
   c. An accumulation of blood under the periosteum, especially of the parietal bones, following labor.
   d. A hemorrhage within the anterior fontanelle.

167. Ophthalmia neonatorum is:
   a. A transitory fever which sometimes occurs in infants during the first days of life.
   b. A highly contagious infection of newborns for which the specific cause is unknown.
   c. A purulent conjunctivitis of the newborn.
   d. Jaundice sometimes seen in the normal newborn infant.

168. Thrush is:
   a. A secretion found in the breast of the newborn infant.
   b. A skin disease caused by staphylococci, characterized by flat vesicles that become pustular.
   c. A disease of infants caused by Candida albicans.
   d. A highly contagious infection of newborns for which the specific cause is unknown.

169. The purpose of genetic counseling is:
   a. To give the parents as much information as is known about the disorder.
   b. To warn parents not to have children.
   c. To enable parents to reach wise decisions.
   d. To inform parents of the recurrence risk of the disorder.
      (1) a is correct.
      (2) b is correct.
      (3) a, b, and d are correct.
      (4) a, c, and d are correct.

170. Which of the following statements apply to sickle cell disease?
   a. Techniques are available to differentiate between those who have sickle cell anemia and those who carry the trait.
   b. A person with sickle cell anemia has inherited a sickle cell gene from each parent.
   c. A person who inherits a sickle cell gene from only one parent is called a trait or carrier.
   d. If only one parent carries the sickle cell trait, two children in four risk inheriting it, and two in four can be expected to be normal.
      (1) a and b are correct.
      (2) a, b, c, and d are correct.
      (3) c and d are correct.
      (4) b and c are correct.